OWEN HUNTER

The Anti-Aging Guide

This book was professionally typeset on Reedsy.
Find out more at reedsy.com

Contents

INTRODUCTION

Unlocking the Secrets to a Longer, Healthier Life

In an age of rapid technological advancement and medical breakthroughs, the quest for longevity has never been more captivating. As we witness the remarkable progress made in fields like regenerative medicine, genetic engineering, and stem cell therapies, the prospect of extending our healthspan and lifespan has become an exciting reality. No longer confined to the realm of science fiction, the ability to slow down, and potentially even reverse, the aging process is now a driving focus for scientists, healthcare practitioners, and individuals alike.

The relentless march of time, however, remains an inescapable truth. Aging, with all its inherent complexities and challenges, is a universal experience that touches the lives of every human being. From the first signs of wrinkles and gray hair to the gradual decline in physical and cognitive capabilities, the aging process can often feel like a formidable adversary, challenging our resilience and our very sense of self.

Yet, amidst this seemingly insurmountable obstacle, a glimmer of hope shines through. The scientific community has made remarkable strides in unraveling the mysteries of aging, identifying the key hallmarks and underlying mechanisms that govern this fundamental biological process. Through groundbreaking research and innovative approaches, we now have a better understanding of how we can harness our own physiology and leverage various lifestyle interventions to combat the ravages of time.

Welcome to "The Anti-Aging Guide" – your comprehensive roadmap to a longer, healthier, and more vibrant life. In the pages that follow, we will embark on an eye-opening journey, exploring the science of aging, the proven strategies for slowing it down, and the emerging therapies that hold the promise of rejuvenation. By arming you with the knowledge and tools necessary to take control of your own aging trajectory, this book aims to empower you to rewrite the narrative of your golden years, transforming them into a time of vitality, fulfillment, and boundless potential.

Understanding the Hallmarks of Aging

At the heart of our pursuit of longevity lies a deeper understanding of the aging process itself. Aging is a complex, multifaceted phenomenon that encompasses a series of interrelated biological changes and cellular adaptations. Over the past decades, scientists have identified nine key hallmarks of aging, which collectively contribute to the gradual deterioration of our bodies and minds.

These hallmarks include genomic instability, telomere attrition, epigenetic alterations, loss of proteostasis, deregulated nutrient sensing, mitochondrial dysfunction, cellular senescence, stem cell exhaustion, and altered intercellular communication. Each of these hallmarks represents a distinct, yet interconnected, facet of the aging process, and addressing them holds the key to unlocking the secrets of longevity.

For instance, genomic instability refers to the accumulation of DNA damage and mutations, which can impair cellular function and lead to the development of age-related diseases. Telomere attrition, the gradual shortening of the protective caps at the ends of our chromosomes, is another hallmark that has been linked to cellular aging and lifespan. Epigenetic alterations, which involve changes in the way our genes are expressed without altering the underlying DNA sequence, can also contribute to the aging phenotype.

As we delve deeper into these hallmarks, we uncover a tapestry of biological processes that work in concert to drive the aging process. By understanding these fundamental mechanisms, we can begin to identify targeted interventions and lifestyle modifications that have the potential to slow down, or even reverse, the effects of aging.

The Power of Lifestyle Choices

While the aging process is largely influenced by our genetic inheritance and the natural passage of time, a growing body of evidence suggests that our lifestyle choices play a crucial role in determining the rate and trajectory of our aging. In fact, recent studies have revealed that up to 70% of an individual's lifespan may be attributed to modifiable lifestyle factors, rather than genetic predisposition alone.

This realization empowers us with the ability to take an active role in shaping our own health and longevity. By making informed choices and adopting evidence-based strategies, we can harness the power of our daily habits to combat the ravages of time and maintain a vibrant, youthful vitality well into our later years.

Throughout this book, we will explore a comprehensive range of lifestyle interventions that have been shown to positively impact the aging process. From optimal nutrition and targeted supplementation to strategic exercise regimens and stress management techniques, each chapter will provide you with practical, science-backed advice to help you build a personalized anti-aging regimen tailored to your unique needs and goals.

By delving into the latest research and best practices, we will uncover the profound influence that factors like diet, physical activity, sleep, and emotional well-being can have on the pace of our aging. Armed with this knowledge, you will be empowered to make informed choices that can significantly enhance your healthspan and lifespan, allowing you to live longer, stronger, and more vibrantly.

The Promise of Emerging Therapies

While the power of lifestyle choices cannot be overstated, the field of anti-aging is also being transformed by the rapid advancements in medical and scientific research. From cutting-edge stem cell therapies to gene-based interventions, the landscape of anti-aging is evolving at an unprecedented pace, offering hope and exciting possibilities for those seeking to defy the ravages of time.

One of the most promising areas of anti-aging research involves the exploration of senescent cells – those that have reached the end of their replicative lifespan and can no longer divide. These cells, while once essential for growth and development, can accumulate over time and contribute to the onset of age-related diseases. Researchers have identified "senolytic" compounds that can selectively eliminate these harmful cells, potentially clearing the way for renewed cellular rejuvenation and tissue regeneration.

Similarly, the field of regenerative medicine, bolstered by the incredible potential of stem cells, holds the promise of reversing the effects of aging. By harnessing the body's natural ability to regenerate and repair damaged tissues, innovative therapies are being developed to address a wide range of age-related conditions, from cognitive decline to cardiovascular disease.

Furthermore, advancements in genetic engineering and epigenetic modulation offer the tantalizing possibility of directly targeting the molecular underpinnings of the aging process. By manipulating the expression of genes and altering the epigenetic landscape, researchers are working to unlock new avenues for longevity and healthspan extension.

As these cutting-edge therapies continue to evolve and gain traction, they will undoubtedly play a crucial role in the future of anti-aging. While some of these interventions may still be in the experimental stage, understanding their potential and keeping abreast of the latest developments will empower you to make informed decisions about your own health and longevity journey.

Embracing the Anti-Aging Mindset

Ultimately, the pursuit of longevity is not just about extending our lifespan, but about enhancing our healthspan – the period of our lives during which we enjoy optimal physical, mental, and emotional well-being. By adopting an anti-aging mindset, we can shift our focus from simply delaying the inevitable to actively embracing a lifestyle that promotes vitality, resilience, and a deep sense of purpose.

This book is designed to be your comprehensive guide to this transformative journey. Within these pages, you will discover a wealth of evidence-based strategies, cutting-edge insights, and practical advice to help you navigate the complex and ever-evolving landscape of anti-aging. Whether you are seeking to maintain your current state of health or looking to reverse the signs of aging, this book will equip you with the knowledge and tools necessary to take control of your own longevity.

As you embark on this journey, remember that the path to a longer, healthier life is not a one-size-fits-all proposition. Each individual's needs and circumstances are unique, and the key lies in finding the right balance of lifestyle interventions, emerging therapies, and personalized approaches that resonate with your own biology, preferences, and goals.

By embracing this anti-aging mindset and actively participating in the ongoing quest for longevity, you will not only unlock the secrets to a longer lifespan but also discover a newfound sense of purpose, vitality, and joy in the years to come. So, let us begin this transformative journey together, and unlock the full potential of a life well-lived.

CHAPTER 1

Introduction to Anti-Aging

As we embark on our journey to unlock the secrets of longevity, it is essential to first understand the fundamental principles that underpin the aging process. In this opening chapter, we will delve into the significance of slowing the aging process, explore the key hallmarks of aging, and lay the groundwork for the comprehensive anti-aging strategies that will be discussed throughout this book.

The Importance of Slowing the Aging Process

Aging is a universal and inevitable experience, one that touches the lives of every human being. From the first appearance of gray hair to the gradual decline in physical and cognitive abilities, the passage of time can often feel like a relentless adversary, challenging our resilience and our very sense of self.

Yet, despite the seemingly inescapable nature of aging, a growing body of scientific evidence suggests that we possess the potential to significantly influence the pace and trajectory of this fundamental biological process. By understanding the underlying mechanisms that drive aging and leveraging the latest advancements in research, we can now take a proactive approach to combating the ravages of time.

The importance of slowing the aging process extends far beyond mere vanity or the desire to maintain a youthful appearance. As we grow older, we face an increased risk of developing a wide range of age-related diseases and conditions, including cancer, cardiovascular disease, neurodegenerative disorders, and type 2 diabetes. These debilitating ailments not only compromise our physical and mental well-being but also have a profound impact on our quality of life, our independence, and our ability to fully engage with the world around us.

By slowing the aging process and maintaining optimal health and vitality, we can potentially delay the onset of these age-related diseases, extend our productive years, and enjoy a more prolonged period of active, fulfilling, and independent living. This, in turn, not only benefits the individual but also has broader societal implications, as it can alleviate the strain on healthcare systems, reduce the burden of long-term care, and enable individuals to remain active contributors to their communities for longer.

Furthermore, the pursuit of longevity is not solely about extending the number of years we live, but about enhancing our "healthspan" – the period of our lives during which we experience optimal physical, mental, and emotional well-being. By adopting an anti-aging mindset and implementing evidence-based strategies, we can strive to achieve a vibrant, energetic, and productive later life, one that is filled with purpose, fulfillment, and the ability to fully engage with the world around us.

The Hallmarks of Aging

At the heart of our understanding of the aging process lies a deeper appreciation for the complex and interconnected biological mechanisms that drive this fundamental phenomenon. Over the past decades, scientists have identified nine key hallmarks of aging, each representing a distinct, yet related, facet of the aging process.

1. Genomic Instability

The first hallmark of aging is genomic instability, which refers to the accumulation of DNA damage and mutations within our cells. As we grow older, our genetic material becomes increasingly susceptible to various types of damage, including single-strand breaks, double-strand breaks, and aberrant epigenetic modifications. These genetic alterations can impair cellular function, compromise cell division, and contribute to the development of age-related diseases, such as cancer and neurodegenerative disorders.

2. Telomere Attrition

Telomeres, the protective caps at the ends of our chromosomes, play a crucial role in maintaining genomic stability and cellular integrity. As we age, these telomeres gradually shorten, a process that has been linked to cellular senescence and the overall aging process. Shorter telomeres are associated with an increased risk of age-related diseases and can serve as a marker of an individual's biological age.

3. Epigenetic Alterations

Epigenetic modifications, which involve changes in gene expression without altering the underlying DNA sequence, are another hallmark of aging. As we grow older, our epigenetic landscape undergoes significant transformations, leading to the dysregulation of important cellular processes. These epigenetic alterations can contribute to the development of age-related diseases, such as Alzheimer's disease and certain types of cancer.

4. Loss of Proteostasis

Proteostasis, the delicate balance between the synthesis, folding, trafficking, and clearance of proteins, is essential for maintaining cellular function and health. However, as we age, this homeostatic mechanism becomes increasingly disrupted, leading to the accumulation of misfolded, damaged, or aggregated proteins. This loss of proteostasis has been linked to a wide range of age-related disorders, including neurodegenerative diseases and metabolic disorders.

5. Deregulated Nutrient Sensing

The ability of our cells to accurately sense and respond to changes in nutrient availability is another hallmark of aging. As we grow older, this nutrient-sensing machinery, which includes pathways like the insulin/IGF-1 signaling and the mechanistic target of rapamycin (mTOR) pathways, becomes deregulated. This can lead to metabolic dysregulation, inflammation, and an increased susceptibility to age-related diseases, such as type 2 diabetes and cardiovascular disease.

6. Mitochondrial Dysfunction

Mitochondria, often referred to as the "powerhouses" of our cells, play a crucial role in energy production and cellular homeostasis. However, as we age, these organelles become increasingly susceptible to damage and dysfunction, leading to reduced energy output, increased oxidative stress, and the potential for further cellular damage and dysfunction.

7. Cellular Senescence

Cellular senescence, the state in which cells have permanently ceased division, is another hallmark of aging. While senescent cells were once essential for growth and development, their accumulation over time can contribute to tissue dysfunction, chronic inflammation, and the development of age-related diseases. Researchers have identified various strategies, such as the use of senolytic compounds, to selectively eliminate these harmful senescent cells.

8. Stem Cell Exhaustion

Stem cells, with their remarkable ability to self-renew and differentiate into various cell types, play a vital role in tissue regeneration and homeostasis. However, as we age, the number and function of these stem cells can become diminished, leading to impaired tissue repair and regeneration, as well as an increased susceptibility to age-related diseases.

9. Altered Intercellular Communication

The final hallmark of aging involves the disruption of intercellular communication, which is essential for the coordination of various physiological processes. As we grow older, the signaling pathways that facilitate communication between cells can become dysregulated, leading to the breakdown of tissue homeostasis and the development of age-related diseases.

Understanding these nine hallmarks of aging is crucial, as they provide a framework for understanding the underlying mechanisms that drive the aging process. By targeting these key aspects of cellular and physiological function, we can begin to develop targeted interventions and comprehensive strategies to slow down the pace of aging and promote optimal health and longevity.

The Multifaceted Nature of Aging

It is important to recognize that the aging process is not a singular, linear phenomenon, but rather a complex, multifaceted, and highly interconnected series of biological changes. The nine hallmarks of aging, while distinct, do not operate in isolation; rather, they interact and influence one another in intricate ways, creating a dynamic and ever-evolving landscape of cellular and organismal aging.

For example, genomic instability can lead to the accumulation of DNA damage, which in turn can trigger epigenetic alterations and disrupt the delicate balance of proteostasis. Similarly, mitochondrial dysfunction can contribute to increased oxidative stress, which can then drive cellular senescence and further exacerbate the deterioration of stem cell function.

This interconnectedness underscores the importance of adopting a holistic, multi-pronged approach to anti-aging interventions. By addressing the aging process at multiple levels, we can leverage the synergistic effects of various strategies to achieve a more profound and lasting impact on our overall health and longevity.

Furthermore, the multifaceted nature of aging also highlights the individualized nature of this process. Each individual's genetic makeup, lifestyle factors, and environmental exposures can contribute to unique patterns of cellular and physiological aging. This emphasizes the need for personalized anti-aging approaches that take into account an individual's specific needs, vulnerabilities, and predispositions.

As we delve deeper into the world of anti-aging, it will become increasingly clear that a one-size-fits-all solution is not the answer. Instead, the key lies in crafting a comprehensive, tailored plan that addresses the multifaceted nature of aging and empowers individuals to take an active role in shaping their own longevity journey.

The Role of Lifestyle Factors

While the aging process is undoubtedly influenced by our genetic makeup and the natural passage of time, a growing body of evidence suggests that our lifestyle choices play a crucial role in determining the rate and trajectory of this fundamental biological phenomenon.

Recent studies have revealed that up to 70% of an individual's lifespan may be attributed to modifiable lifestyle factors, rather than genetic predisposition alone. This realization empowers us with the ability to take an active role in shaping our own health and longevity, as we can leverage the power of our daily habits and behaviors to combat the ravages of time.

Throughout this book, we will explore a comprehensive range of lifestyle interventions that have been shown to positively impact the aging process. From optimal nutrition and targeted supplementation to strategic exercise regimens and stress management techniques, each chapter will provide you with practical, science-backed advice to help you build a personalized anti-aging regimen tailored to your unique needs and goals.

By delving into the latest research and best practices, we will uncover the profound influence that factors like diet, physical activity, sleep, and emotional well-being can have on the pace of our aging. Armed with this knowledge, you will be empowered to make informed choices that can significantly enhance your healthspan and lifespan, allowing you to live longer, stronger, and more vibrantly.

The Power of Lifestyle Choices

One of the most impactful lifestyle factors in the context of anti-aging is nutrition. The foods we consume, the way we nourish our bodies, can have a profound effect on the cellular and physiological processes that underpin the aging process. By adopting an anti-aging dietary approach that emphasizes nutrient-dense, whole foods, we can harness the power of essential macronutrients, micronutrients, and phytochemicals to support cellular health, reduce oxidative stress, and promote longevity.

Similarly, regular physical activity has been shown to be a powerful tool in the fight against aging. From strength training to cardiovascular exercise, strategic movement can help maintain muscle mass, improve cardiovascular function, boost cognitive abilities, and even enhance stem cell function – all of which are crucial for slowing the aging process and preserving our overall health and vitality.

The role of stress management and emotional well-being is another important consideration in the realm of anti-aging. Chronic stress, whether physical or psychological, can have a detrimental impact on our cellular and physiological processes, contributing to inflammation, accelerated cellular aging, and an increased risk of age-related diseases. By incorporating stress-reducing techniques, such as mindfulness, meditation, and relaxation practices, we can mitigate the harmful effects of stress and foster a state of emotional balance and resilience.

Furthermore, the quality and quantity of our sleep can also play a pivotal role in the aging process. Adequate, high-quality sleep is essential for cellular repair, hormonal regulation, and the maintenance of healthy cognitive function. By optimizing our sleep habits and aligning our circadian rhythms, we can support the body's natural rejuvenation processes and enhance our overall longevity.

These are just a few examples of the powerful lifestyle factors that can shape the trajectory of our aging. Throughout this book, we will delve deeper into each of these areas, providing you with the knowledge and tools necessary to create a comprehensive anti-aging plan that addresses the multifaceted nature of this fundamental biological process.

Embracing the Anti-Aging Mindset

As we embark on this journey to unlock the secrets of longevity, it is essential to cultivate an anti-aging mindset – a holistic, proactive approach to maintaining and enhancing our health and well-being as we grow older.

This mindset shift goes beyond simply delaying the inevitable; it is about embracing a lifestyle that promotes vitality, resilience, and a deep sense of purpose. It is about recognizing that our later years need not be defined by decline, but can instead be a time of renewed energy, fulfillment, and the ability to fully engage with the world around us.

By adopting this anti-aging mindset, we can shift our focus from treating age-related diseases to actively preventing them, from passively accepting the ravages of time to actively shaping our own longevity trajectory. This empowered perspective will serve as the foundation for the comprehensive strategies and interventions that will be explored throughout this book.

As you embark on this transformative journey, remember that the path to a longer, healthier life is not a one-size-fits-all proposition. Each individual's needs and circumstances are unique, and the key lies in finding the right balance of lifestyle interventions, emerging therapies, and personalized approaches that resonate with your own biology, preferences, and goals.

By embracing this anti-aging mindset and actively participating in the ongoing quest for longevity, you will not only unlock the secrets to a longer lifespan but also discover a newfound sense of purpose, vitality, and joy in the years to come. So, let us begin this transformative journey together, and unlock the full potential of a life well-lived.

CHAPTER 2

Nutrition for Longevity

In the pursuit of longevity, one of the most powerful tools at our disposal is the food we choose to nourish our bodies. The field of nutritional science has made remarkable strides in understanding the pivotal role that diet plays in the aging process, unveiling a wealth of insights that can empower us to take control of our own longevity journey.

In this chapter, we will delve into the intricate relationship between nutrition and anti-aging, exploring the vital roles that macronutrients, micronutrients, and various dietary patterns play in supporting cellular health, reducing oxidative stress, and promoting overall longevity.

The Role of Macronutrients in Anti-Aging

Macronutrients, the three main components of our diet (protein, carbohydrates, and fats), are not only essential for maintaining our overall health and well-being, but they also hold the key to unlocking the secrets of longevity.

Protein: The Building Blocks of Rejuvenation

Protein is a macronutrient that is essential for the growth, repair, and maintenance of our body's tissues and organs. As we age, the body's ability to efficiently utilize and synthesize protein can diminish, leading to the gradual loss of muscle mass (sarcopenia) and the impairment of various physiological processes.

However, by ensuring an adequate intake of high-quality, protein-rich foods, we can combat this age-related decline and support the body's natural rejuvenation processes. Protein sources such as lean meats, poultry, fish, eggs, dairy, and plant-based options like legumes, nuts, and seeds, provide the essential amino acids necessary for the repair and regeneration of cells, the maintenance of muscle mass, and the support of immune function.

Furthermore, research has shown that higher protein intake, particularly from plant-based sources, can have a positive impact on longevity by reducing the risk of age-related diseases, such as cardiovascular disease, type 2 diabetes, and certain types of cancer.

Carbohydrates: Fueling the Fires of Longevity

Carbohydrates, the body's primary source of energy, play a crucial role in supporting the various physiological processes that underpin the aging process. However, not all carbohydrates are created equal, and the type and quality of carbohydrates we consume can have a significant impact on our longevity.

Whole, fiber-rich carbohydrates, such as those found in fruits, vegetables, whole grains, and legumes, have been associated with numerous anti-aging benefits. These nutrient-dense carbohydrates can help regulate blood sugar levels, reduce inflammation, and support a healthy gut microbiome – all of which are essential for maintaining optimal health and longevity.

In contrast, refined and processed carbohydrates, which are often high in added sugars and lack the beneficial fiber and nutrients, can contribute to the development of age-related diseases, such as type 2 diabetes, cardiovascular disease, and cognitive decline. By prioritizing whole, complex carbohydrates and limiting the intake of refined and processed options, we can leverage the power of this macronutrient to support our longevity goals.

Fats: The Healthy Allies in Anti-Aging

Fats, the third macronutrient, have long been a topic of debate in the realm of health and nutrition. However, emerging research has shed light on the vital role that certain fats play in the anti-aging process.

Unsaturated fats, particularly the omega-3 fatty acids found in foods like fatty fish, nuts, and seeds, have been shown to possess potent anti-inflammatory properties. Inflammation is a key driver of the aging process, contributing to the development of various age-related diseases. By incorporating these healthy fats into our diets, we can help mitigate the detrimental effects of inflammation and support overall cellular and physiological function.

Additionally, fats play a crucial role in the absorption and utilization of fat-soluble vitamins, such as vitamins A, D, E, and K, which are essential for a wide range of anti-aging processes, from maintaining skin health to supporting bone density and cognitive function.

While it is important to consume fats in moderation and to prioritize the intake of unsaturated over saturated and trans fats, adopting a balanced approach to this macronutrient can contribute to the promotion of longevity and the preservation of our overall health and well-being.

Micronutrients and Antioxidants for Cellular Health

Beyond the macronutrients that provide the foundational building blocks for our bodies, the micronutrients and antioxidants found in our diets also play a vital role in supporting the anti-aging process.

Vitamins and Minerals: The Essential Cofactors for Longevity

Vitamins and minerals, collectively known as micronutrients, are required in smaller quantities compared to macronutrients, but their importance cannot be overstated. These essential nutrients serve as cofactors for a myriad of cellular processes, from energy production to DNA repair and cellular regeneration.

For example, vitamin C is a powerful antioxidant that can help neutralize free radicals and support the immune system, while vitamin E protects cell membranes from oxidative damage. Minerals like zinc, selenium, and magnesium are also crucial for maintaining optimal cellular function and supporting the body's natural defenses against the ravages of time.

By ensuring an adequate intake of a wide variety of micronutrient-rich foods, such as fruits, vegetables, whole grains, and lean proteins, we can harness the synergistic benefits of these essential nutrients to promote longevity and combat the effects of aging.

Antioxidants: The Guardians of Cellular Health

Antioxidants, both those produced naturally within the body and those obtained through our diet, play a pivotal role in the anti-aging process. These powerful compounds are responsible for neutralizing harmful free radicals and reactive oxygen species, which can cause significant damage to cellular structures, DNA, and proteins.

The accumulation of oxidative stress is a hallmark of the aging process, contributing to the development of a wide range of age-related diseases, including cancer, cardiovascular disease, and neurodegenerative disorders. By incorporating antioxidant-rich foods into our diets, we can help mitigate the detrimental effects of oxidative stress and support the body's natural ability to maintain cellular integrity and function.

Some of the most well-known and potent dietary antioxidants include vitamins C and E, carotenoids like lycopene and beta-carotene, and polyphenols found in fruits, vegetables, tea, and cocoa. By diversifying our intake of these antioxidant-rich foods, we can create a powerful synergy that enhances our cellular defenses and promotes longevity.

Dietary Strategies for Extending Lifespan

While the roles of macronutrients and micronutrients in the anti-aging process are undoubtedly crucial, the way we combine and integrate these dietary elements can also have a significant impact on our longevity.

The Mediterranean Diet: A Longevity-Promoting Approach

The Mediterranean diet, a plant-based dietary pattern that has been heavily studied for its health benefits, has emerged as a particularly promising approach for promoting longevity and combating the effects of aging.

This dietary pattern, which is typically characterized by a high intake of fruits, vegetables, whole grains, legumes, nuts, and olive oil, as well as moderate consumption of fish and dairy, has been associated with a reduced risk of various age-related diseases, including cardiovascular disease, type 2 diabetes, and certain types of cancer.

The key to the Mediterranean diet's anti-aging effects lies in its ability to provide a balanced, nutrient-dense source of macronutrients and micronutrients, while also incorporating beneficial bioactive compounds like polyphenols and omega-3 fatty acids. This synergistic combination supports a wide range of cellular and physiological processes, from reducing inflammation to enhancing mitochondrial function and promoting healthy aging.

Furthermore, the Mediterranean diet's emphasis on plant-based foods and the moderate consumption of animal-based products, such as red meat, can also contribute to its longevity-promoting benefits. This approach helps to maintain a healthy balance of nutrient intake, while also limiting the intake of potentially pro-inflammatory or pro-oxidant compounds that can accelerate the aging process.

By adopting a Mediterranean-inspired dietary approach, individuals can leverage the power of whole, nutrient-dense foods to support their anti-aging goals and improve their overall health and well-being.

Calorie Restriction: A Proven Longevity Intervention

Another dietary strategy that has gained significant attention in the field of anti-aging is calorie restriction. This approach, which involves a moderate reduction in the overall caloric intake (typically by 10-30%), has been consistently shown to extend lifespan and healthspan in a wide range of animal models, from rodents to non-human primates.

The mechanisms behind calorie restriction's anti-aging effects are multifaceted and involve a complex interplay of cellular and physiological adaptations. By reducing the overall caloric intake, the body enters a state of mild stress, which can trigger a cascade of beneficial responses, including reduced oxidative stress, enhanced cellular repair mechanisms, and improved metabolic efficiency.

Calorie restriction has been linked to a decreased risk of age-related diseases, such as cardiovascular disease, cancer, and neurodegenerative disorders. Additionally, this dietary approach has been shown to positively impact various hallmarks of aging, including genomic stability, proteostasis, and mitochondrial function.

While the implementation of a calorie-restricted diet can be challenging for some individuals, various fasting-mimicking protocols, such as intermittent fasting and time-restricted eating, have emerged as more accessible and sustainable alternatives. These approaches can help individuals leverage the benefits of calorie restriction without the need for drastic, long-term reductions in food intake.

It is important to note that the adoption of any calorie-restricted or fasting-based dietary strategy should be done under the guidance of a healthcare professional, particularly for individuals with underlying medical conditions or those taking certain medications.

Personalized Nutrition for Longevity

As we delve deeper into the realm of anti-aging nutrition, it becomes increasingly clear that a one-size-fits-all approach is not the answer. Each individual's genetic makeup, lifestyle factors, and unique physiological characteristics can contribute to distinct patterns of cellular aging and nutrient requirements.

Personalized nutrition, which involves the tailoring of dietary interventions based on an individual's specific needs and predispositions, has emerged as a promising strategy for promoting longevity. By leveraging the power of nutrigenomics, epigenetics, and advanced biomarker analysis, healthcare professionals can now develop customized dietary plans that address the unique drivers of aging for each individual.

This personalized approach to anti-aging nutrition may involve the optimization of macronutrient ratios, the targeted supplementation of specific micronutrients, the incorporation of prebiotics and probiotics to support gut health, and the implementation of tailored fasting or calorie-restricted protocols.

Furthermore, as our understanding of the human gut microbiome continues to evolve, the role of personalized nutrition in shaping the composition and diversity of this vital microbial ecosystem has become increasingly recognized. By nourishing the gut with the right balance of nutrients, we can foster a healthy, resilient microbiome that can positively influence a wide range of physiological processes, from immune function to cognitive performance.

By embracing the power of personalized nutrition, individuals can take a proactive and targeted approach to combating the effects of aging, leveraging the unique characteristics of their own biology to achieve optimal longevity and overall health.

Supplementation and Nutraceuticals

While a nutrient-dense, whole-food-based diet should serve as the foundation of any anti-aging nutritional strategy, the strategic use of dietary supplements and nutraceuticals can also play a valuable role in supporting longevity.

Dietary Supplements for Longevity

Dietary supplements, which can include vitamins, minerals, herbs, and other bioactive compounds, can provide a targeted means of addressing specific nutritional gaps or deficiencies that may arise as we age.

For example, supplements containing omega-3 fatty acids, such as fish oil or krill oil, can help offset the age-related decline in the body's production of these essential fats, which are crucial for maintaining cardiovascular health, reducing inflammation, and supporting cognitive function.

Similarly, antioxidant-rich supplements, like those containing vitamins C and E, carotenoids, or polyphenols, can help bolster the body's defenses against oxidative stress and support cellular integrity.

It is important to note, however, that the use of dietary supplements should be approached with caution and in consultation with a healthcare professional. Some supplements can interact with medications or have potential side effects, particularly when consumed in high doses or without a clear understanding of an individual's specific needs and health status.

Nutraceuticals: The Intersection of Nutrition and Pharmaceuticals

Nutraceuticals, a term that combines "nutrition" and "pharmaceuticals," refer to a category of products that exist at the intersection of food and medicine. These substances, which may include plant-derived compounds, fermentation products, or even synthetic molecules, are designed to provide targeted therapeutic benefits beyond basic nutrition.

In the realm of anti-aging, certain nutraceuticals have shown promising potential in addressing the hallmarks of aging and promoting longevity. For example, compounds like resveratrol, found in red wine and certain berries, have been studied for their ability to activate longevity-promoting pathways, such as the SIRT1 gene, and support mitochondrial function.

Another example is the nutraceutical compound metformin, which is primarily used to manage type 2 diabetes but has also been explored for its potential anti-aging properties. Metformin has been shown to positively impact various hallmarks of aging, including deregulated nutrient sensing, cellular senescence, and stem cell exhaustion.

As with dietary supplements, the use of nutraceuticals should be carefully considered and discussed with a healthcare professional, as these products may have specific dosing requirements, potential side effects, or interactions with medications or other health conditions.

Embracing the Power of Nutritional Interventions

In the pursuit of longevity, the power of nutrition cannot be overstated. By thoughtfully incorporating the principles of macronutrient balance, micronutrient optimization, and targeted supplementation, individuals can leverage the synergistic benefits of these dietary interventions to combat the effects of aging and promote overall health and well-being.

As you embark on this anti-aging journey, remember that the key lies in adopting a holistic, personalized approach to nutrition. By considering your unique genetic makeup, lifestyle factors, and health status, you can create a customized dietary plan that addresses the specific drivers of aging within your own body.

Whether it's embracing the Mediterranean diet, exploring the benefits of calorie restriction, or selectively incorporating targeted supplements and nutraceuticals, the choices you make in the kitchen can have a profound impact on the longevity and quality of your golden years.

By empowering yourself with the knowledge and tools presented in this chapter, you can take an active role in shaping your own aging trajectory, unlocking the secrets to a longer, healthier, and more vibrant life. So, let us continue our journey, one delicious and nutritious bite at a time.

CHAPTER 3

Exercise and Fitness for Anti-Aging

In the pursuit of longevity, the importance of physical activity and fitness cannot be overstated. Emerging research has shed light on the profound impact that strategic exercise can have on the aging process, revealing a powerful arsenal of tools that can be leveraged to slow down the clock and maintain optimal health and vitality well into our golden years.

In this chapter, we will explore the myriad benefits of regular physical activity, delving into the specific ways in which exercise can positively influence the hallmarks of aging. From the preservation of muscle mass to the enhancement of cardiovascular function and cognitive performance, we will uncover the transformative power of an active lifestyle in the fight against the ravages of time.

The Benefits of Regular Physical Activity

As we age, our bodies undergo a gradual decline in physical function, a process that can be significantly slowed down through the adoption of a consistent exercise regimen. By engaging in a well-rounded fitness routine, individuals can harness the power of movement to maintain their independence, improve their quality of life, and stave off the onset of age-related diseases.

Preserving Muscle Mass and Strength

One of the most profound impacts of exercise on the aging process is its ability to maintain and even enhance muscle mass and strength. This is a critical consideration, as the natural decline in muscle mass and strength, a condition known as sarcopenia, is a hallmark of aging that can significantly impair physical function, mobility, and overall quality of life.

Through resistance training, such as weightlifting or bodyweight exercises, individuals can stimulate the growth and maintenance of muscle fibers, counteracting the age-related loss of lean muscle mass. This, in turn, can improve physical performance, increase bone density, and support the body's ability to perform everyday tasks with ease.

Moreover, the preservation of muscle mass and strength can have a cascading effect on other aspects of health. By maintaining a robust musculoskeletal system, individuals can reduce their risk of falls and fractures, which are a major concern for older adults. Additionally, the maintenance of muscle mass has been linked to improved metabolic function, better glycemic control, and a decreased risk of chronic diseases like type 2 diabetes.

Enhancing Cardiovascular Function

Alongside the preservation of muscle mass, regular cardiovascular exercise plays a vital role in supporting healthy aging. As we grow older, our cardiovascular system undergoes a gradual decline, with factors such as stiffening of the arteries, reduced heart pumping capacity, and impaired blood vessel function contributing to an increased risk of cardiovascular disease.

However, by engaging in regular aerobic activities, such as brisk walking, cycling, swimming, or jogging, individuals can improve their cardiovascular fitness and mitigate the age-related deterioration of their heart and blood vessels. This can lead to a host of anti-aging benefits, including:

- Improved blood pressure regulation

- Enhanced endothelial function (the health of the inner lining of blood vessels)
  - Increased oxygen delivery to tissues
  - Reduced inflammation and oxidative stress
  - Better glucose and lipid metabolism

By maintaining a robust cardiovascular system, individuals can not only reduce their risk of heart disease, stroke, and other age-related conditions but also support the overall health and function of their bodies, allowing them to remain active and independent for longer.

Promoting Cognitive Function and Brain Health

In addition to its physical benefits, regular exercise has also been shown to have a profound impact on cognitive function and brain health as we age. The aging process is often accompanied by a gradual decline in cognitive abilities, including memory, attention, and processing speed, which can significantly impact an individual's quality of life and independence.

However, numerous studies have demonstrated that regular physical activity can help offset this age-related cognitive decline. Aerobic exercise, in particular, has been linked to the following brain-boosting benefits:

- Increased blood flow and oxygen delivery to the brain
  - Stimulation of neurogenesis (the growth of new brain cells)
  - Enhanced synaptic plasticity (the ability of brain cells to form new connections)
  - Improved executive function, such as planning, problem-solving, and decision-making
  - Reduced risk of neurodegenerative diseases like Alzheimer's and Parkinson's

Furthermore, the cognitive benefits of exercise extend beyond just the aging brain. Regular physical activity has also been shown to improve mood, reduce stress and anxiety, and promote better sleep – all of which are crucial for maintaining optimal brain health and cognitive function throughout the lifespan.

By prioritizing a fitness routine that includes a combination of cardiovascular, strength, and cognitive-enhancing exercises, individuals can take a proactive approach to safeguarding their brain health and preserving their mental acuity as they grow older.

Strengthening the Immune System

As we age, the human immune system undergoes significant changes, often leading to a weakened response to infections and a decreased ability to fight off harmful pathogens. This age-related decline in immune function, known as immunosenescence, can leave older adults more vulnerable to infectious diseases, autoimmune disorders, and even certain types of cancer.

Remarkably, regular physical activity has been shown to have a positive impact on the aging immune system. Exercise can help stimulate the production and function of various immune cells, such as T cells, B cells, and natural killer cells, while also reducing systemic inflammation – a key driver of immunosenescence.

Additionally, exercise has been linked to improved vaccine response in older adults, enhancing their ability to mount a robust and protective immune response to various infectious agents. By maintaining a physically active lifestyle, individuals can help bolster their immune defenses and reduce their susceptibility to age-related immune dysfunction.

Fostering a Healthier Gut Microbiome

The gut microbiome, the trillions of microorganisms that reside within our gastrointestinal tract, has emerged as a crucial player in the aging process. As we grow older, the composition and diversity of our gut microbiome can become imbalanced, contributing to the development of various age-related conditions, such as inflammatory bowel diseases, metabolic disorders, and even neurodegenerative diseases.

Interestingly, regular physical activity has been shown to have a positive impact on the gut microbiome, promoting a more diverse and resilient microbial ecosystem. Exercise can influence the gut microbiome in several ways, including:

- Increasing the production of short-chain fatty acids, which support gut barrier function and immune regulation
   - Modulating the expression of genes involved in gut barrier integrity and inflammation
   - Altering the relative abundance of beneficial bacterial species, such as Bifidobacterium and Lactobacillus

By maintaining an active lifestyle, individuals can help foster a healthier, more balanced gut microbiome, which in turn can support various physiological processes and reduce the risk of age-related diseases.

Harnessing the Power of Strategic Exercise

With a deeper understanding of the multifaceted benefits of regular physical activity, the next step is to explore the specific exercise strategies and regimens that can be most effectively leveraged to combat the aging process.

Strength Training and Muscle Maintenance
   As previously discussed, the preservation of muscle mass and strength is a critical component of successful aging. To this end, strength training exercises, such as weightlifting, resistance band training, and bodyweight exercises, should be a cornerstone of any anti-aging fitness routine.

These types of exercises work by challenging the muscles to overcome resistance, which triggers a series of adaptations that lead to the growth and maintenance of muscle fibers. By incorporating strength training into their weekly routine, individuals can not only combat the age-related loss of muscle mass but also improve their physical function, balance, and overall quality of life.

When designing a strength training program for anti-aging, it is important to consider the following principles:

- Progression: Gradually increase the intensity, volume, and complexity of exercises over time to continually challenge the muscles.
  - Compound movements: Focus on exercises that engage multiple muscle groups simultaneously, such as squats, deadlifts, and push-ups.
  - Varied grip positions: Incorporate different grip widths and hand positions to target the muscles from different angles.
  - Adequate rest and recovery: Allow for sufficient rest between strength training sessions to facilitate muscle repair and growth.

By adhering to these principles and tailoring the strength training regimen to their individual needs and abilities, individuals can optimize the anti-aging benefits of this essential exercise modality.

Cardiovascular Exercise and Cardiovascular Health

In addition to strength training, regular cardiovascular exercise is a crucial component of any comprehensive anti-aging fitness strategy. Engaging in activities that elevate the heart rate, such as brisk walking, jogging, cycling, swimming, or dancing, can have a profound impact on cardiovascular function and overall health.

Cardiovascular exercise has been shown to improve the following markers of cardiovascular health:

- Resting heart rate: Lower resting heart rate is associated with improved cardiovascular efficiency.

- Blood pressure: Regular exercise can help lower both systolic and diastolic blood pressure.
- Endothelial function: Exercise can enhance the ability of blood vessels to dilate and improve blood flow.
- Cholesterol levels: Cardiovascular exercise can help lower LDL (bad) cholesterol and increase HDL (good) cholesterol.

By incorporating cardiovascular exercise into their weekly routine, individuals can not only reduce their risk of age-related cardiovascular diseases but also support the overall health and resilience of their cardiovascular system.

When designing a cardiovascular exercise program for anti-aging, it is important to consider factors such as:

- Intensity: Moderate-to-vigorous intensity exercises, such as brisk walking or jogging, are typically recommended for optimal cardiovascular benefits.
- Duration: Aim for at least 150 minutes of moderate-intensity or 75 minutes of vigorous-intensity exercise per week.
- Variety: Incorporate a mix of different cardiovascular activities to keep the body challenged and engaged.

Remember, the key to success is to find activities that you enjoy and can consistently incorporate into your lifestyle, as adherence is crucial for reaping the long-term anti-aging benefits of cardiovascular exercise.

Cognitive-Enhancing Exercises

While physical exercise is essential for maintaining muscle strength, cardiovascular health, and overall physical function, it is also crucial to incorporate activities that specifically target cognitive function and brain health as we age.

Exercises that challenge the mind and promote neuroplasticity, the brain's ability to adapt and form new connections, can have a profound impact on cognitive performance and help offset age-related cognitive decline.

Some examples of cognitive-enhancing exercises include:

- Coordinative exercises: Activities that require the coordination of multiple body parts, such as dance, tai chi, or juggling, can stimulate the brain and enhance executive function.
  - Cognitive training: Engaging in activities that challenge the mind, such as puzzles, memory games, or learning a new skill, can help improve cognitive flexibility and processing speed.
  - Dual-task training: Performing physical and cognitive tasks simultaneously, such as walking while solving a mental problem, can improve multitasking abilities and overall cognitive function.

By incorporating a mix of these cognitive-enhancing exercises into their fitness routine, individuals can support the health and resilience of their brain, promoting better memory, attention, and problem-solving skills as they age.

Integrating Exercise into a Comprehensive Anti-Aging Lifestyle

While the benefits of regular exercise in the context of anti-aging are clear, it is important to recognize that physical activity should be just one component of a comprehensive, holistic approach to longevity. By integrating exercise into a broader lifestyle that addresses other key factors, such as nutrition, stress management, and sleep, individuals can amplify the anti-aging benefits and achieve optimal health and vitality.

For example, coupling a regular exercise routine with a nutrient-dense, anti-inflammatory diet can help support the body's cellular repair processes, reduce oxidative stress, and promote overall metabolic health. Similarly, incorporating stress-management techniques, such as meditation or yoga, can help mitigate the detrimental effects of chronic stress on the aging process.

Furthermore, ensuring adequate, high-quality sleep is crucial for allowing the body to fully recover and rejuvenate from the stresses of daily life and exercise. By aligning exercise with other healthy lifestyle habits, individuals can create a synergistic effect that enhances their overall resilience and slows down the pace of aging.

When developing a personalized anti-aging fitness plan, it is essential to consider individual factors such as age, current fitness level, any pre-existing health conditions, and personal preferences. A one-size-fits-all approach is not effective, as the optimal exercise regimen may vary significantly from person to person.

By working closely with healthcare professionals, such as physical therapists, personal trainers, or exercise physiologists, individuals can create a tailored exercise program that addresses their unique needs and goals. This individualized approach can help ensure the safety, effectiveness, and sustainability of the exercise routine, allowing individuals to reap the full benefits of physical activity in their quest for longevity.

Embracing the Transformative Power of Exercise

As we have explored in this chapter, regular physical activity is a powerful tool in the fight against the ravages of time. By harnessing the benefits of strength training, cardiovascular exercise, and cognitive-enhancing activities, individuals can combat the age-related decline in physical and cognitive function, promote overall health and resilience, and unlock the secrets to a longer, more vibrant life.

However, the true transformative power of exercise lies not only in its ability to improve physical and cognitive outcomes but also in its capacity to instill a profound sense of empowerment and self-determination. By taking an active role in shaping their own aging trajectory through the adoption of a comprehensive fitness routine, individuals can reclaim control over their health and well-being, fostering a deep sense of purpose and vitality that can permeate every aspect of their lives.

As you embark on this anti-aging journey, remember that the path to longevity is not a solitary one. By surrounding yourself with a supportive network of healthcare professionals, exercise enthusiasts, and like-minded individuals, you can cultivate a community of accountability, motivation, and shared experiences that will further propel you towards your goals.

Embrace the challenge, celebrate the small victories, and never lose sight of the transformative power that lies within your own body and mind. Through the consistent and mindful practice of exercise, you hold the key to unlocking a future filled with boundless energy, vibrant health, and the boundless joy of a life well-lived.

CHAPTER 4

Stress Management and Emotional Well-being

As we navigate the complex landscape of anti-aging, it becomes increasingly clear that our physical health is intrinsically linked to our emotional and psychological well-being. Stress, a pervasive aspect of modern life, can have a profound and insidious impact on the aging process, contributing to the development of a wide range of age-related diseases and undermining our overall longevity.

In this chapter, we will explore the critical role that stress management and the cultivation of emotional well-being play in the quest for a longer, healthier life. By delving into the science behind the mind-body connection, we will uncover the powerful ways in which our thoughts, emotions, and relationships can shape the trajectory of our aging journey.

The Impact of Stress on Aging

Stress, a physiological and psychological response to perceived threats or challenges, is a universal human experience. However, when stress becomes chronic and persistent, it can have a detrimental impact on our physical and mental health, accelerating the aging process and increasing our susceptibility to a host of age-related conditions.

At the heart of this stress-aging connection lies the body's intricate stress response system, known as the hypothalamic-pituitary-adrenal (HPA) axis. When we encounter a stressful situation, this system is activated, triggering the release of hormones like cortisol, which help the body mount an appropriate response.

While this stress response is an essential adaptive mechanism, designed to help us cope with and overcome challenges, the constant activation of the HPA axis due to chronic stress can have a profoundly negative impact on our health and longevity. Some of the key ways in which stress can accelerate the aging process include:

1. Increased Oxidative Stress and Inflammation
   Chronic stress has been shown to increase the production of free radicals and reactive oxygen species, leading to heightened oxidative stress within the body. This, in turn, can cause damage to cellular structures, DNA, and proteins, contributing to the development of age-related diseases, such as cardiovascular disease, cancer, and neurodegenerative disorders.

Furthermore, stress is a potent driver of inflammation, a hallmark of the aging process that has been linked to a wide range of health problems. The sustained release of inflammatory mediators like cytokines can disrupt the body's delicate balance, leading to chronic low-grade inflammation and exacerbating the aging process.

2. Accelerated Telomere Shortening
   Telomeres, the protective caps at the ends of our chromosomes, play a crucial role in cellular aging. As we grow older, these telomeres gradually shorten, a process that has been associated with an increased risk of age-related diseases. Interestingly, research has shown that chronic stress can accelerate telomere shortening, potentially hastening the onset of cellular senescence and the associated health consequences.

3. Disruption of Hormonal Balance

Stress can have a significant impact on the body's endocrine system, leading to imbalances in critical hormones that are essential for maintaining optimal health and longevity. For example, the sustained elevation of cortisol can disrupt the delicate balance of sex hormones, such as estrogen and testosterone, as well as hormones that regulate metabolism, sleep, and immune function.

These hormonal imbalances can contribute to a wide range of age-related conditions, including metabolic disorders, sexual dysfunction, and cognitive decline, further undermining an individual's overall well-being and quality of life.

4. Impaired Immune Function

Chronic stress has been shown to compromise the immune system, impairing the body's ability to mount an effective defense against pathogens and contributing to the development of age-related immune dysfunction, or immunosenescence.

The sustained activation of the stress response can lead to the dysregulation of immune cells, such as T cells and natural killer cells, as well as the overproduction of inflammatory cytokines. This, in turn, can increase the risk of infections, autoimmune disorders, and certain types of cancer, all of which are more prevalent in older adults.

5. Cognitive Decline and Neurodegeneration

The impact of stress on the brain is particularly concerning in the context of aging. Chronic stress has been linked to the accelerated loss of brain volume, particularly in regions associated with memory and cognitive function, such as the hippocampus and prefrontal cortex.

Furthermore, stress-induced inflammation and the overproduction of damaging molecules, like free radicals, can contribute to the development of neurodegenerative diseases, such as Alzheimer's and Parkinson's, as well as the general decline in cognitive abilities that often accompanies the aging process.

Cultivating Emotional Well-being and Stress Resilience

Given the profound and multifaceted impact of stress on the aging process, the importance of developing effective stress management strategies and cultivating emotional well-being cannot be overstated. By adopting a holistic approach to mental and emotional health, individuals can not only mitigate the detrimental effects of stress but also unlock the vast potential for longevity and vitality.

Mindfulness and Meditation: The Path to Stress Reduction

At the forefront of the anti-stress arsenal lies the practice of mindfulness and meditation. These ancient contemplative practices have gained significant attention in recent years for their ability to reduce stress, promote emotional regulation, and enhance overall well-being.

Mindfulness, the act of being present and fully attentive to the current moment, has been shown to have a profound impact on the body's stress response. By training the mind to observe thoughts and emotions without judgment or reactivity, individuals can effectively interrupt the cycle of rumination and stress-induced physiological activation, leading to a greater sense of calm and control.

Numerous studies have demonstrated the benefits of mindfulness and meditation in the context of anti-aging. These practices have been linked to:

- Reduced cortisol levels and improved regulation of the HPA axis
    - Enhanced telomerase activity, which can help maintain telomere length
    - Decreased inflammation and oxidative stress
    - Improved immune function and resilience
    - Enhanced cognitive performance and reduced risk of neurodegeneration

By incorporating mindfulness-based techniques, such as focused breathing exercises, body scans, or guided imagery, into their daily routines, individuals can cultivate a greater sense of inner calm and emotional stability, effectively buffering themselves against the ravages of chronic stress.

Fostering Positive Emotions and Relationships

In addition to the power of mindfulness and meditation, the cultivation of positive emotions and healthy relationships can also play a pivotal role in the pursuit of longevity and well-being.

Emerging research has highlighted the profound impact that positive emotions, such as joy, gratitude, and compassion, can have on the aging process. These emotional states have been associated with a wide range of health benefits, including:

- Reduced inflammation and oxidative stress
    - Improved cardiovascular function and metabolic health
    - Enhanced immune function and resilience
    - Increased neuroplasticity and cognitive performance
    - Improved overall subjective well-being and life satisfaction

By actively cultivating and nurturing positive emotions through practices like gratitude journaling, acts of kindness, or savoring meaningful experiences, individuals can create a powerful synergy between their mental and physical health, unlocking the secrets to a longer, more vibrant life.

Furthermore, the quality and depth of our social relationships have also been identified as crucial factors in the anti-aging equation. Strong, supportive social connections have been linked to a reduced risk of age-related diseases, improved cognitive function, and enhanced emotional well-being.

Conversely, social isolation and loneliness have been identified as significant risk factors for a host of age-related conditions, including cardiovascular disease, cognitive decline, and depression. By actively fostering and maintaining meaningful relationships with family, friends, and communities, individuals can build a supportive network that can help them navigate the challenges of aging with resilience and optimism.

Stress Management Techniques for Optimal Longevity

While the cultivation of mindfulness, positive emotions, and healthy relationships are essential pillars of a comprehensive stress management strategy, there are a variety of other techniques and practices that can further enhance an individual's ability to manage stress and promote longevity.

Relaxation Practices

Incorporating relaxation practices, such as deep breathing exercises, progressive muscle relaxation, or guided imagery, can help activate the body's parasympathetic nervous system, which is responsible for the "rest and digest" response. These practices have been shown to reduce physiological markers of stress, like heart rate and blood pressure, while also promoting a sense of calm and well-being.

Regular practice of these relaxation techniques can help individuals better manage the physical and psychological manifestations of stress, enabling them to maintain a state of equilibrium and resilience in the face of life's challenges.

Physical Activity and Exercise

As discussed in the previous chapter, regular physical activity and exercise not only benefit the body's physical health but also play a crucial role in managing stress and promoting emotional well-being.

Engaging in aerobic exercise, strength training, or even gentle movement practices like yoga or tai chi can help reduce stress by:

- Increasing the production of mood-boosting neurotransmitters, such as

endorphins and serotonin
- Decreasing the body's physiological stress response, including reduced cortisol levels
- Improving sleep quality, which is essential for stress recovery and emotional regulation
- Enhancing self-efficacy and feelings of accomplishment, which can boost confidence and resilience

By seamlessly integrating physical activity into their anti-aging lifestyle, individuals can create a powerful synergy between their physical and mental health, further strengthening their resilience to the ravages of stress.

Sleep Optimization
The importance of quality sleep in the context of stress management and longevity cannot be overstated. Adequate, restorative sleep is essential for allowing the body and mind to recover from the daily stresses of life, as well as for supporting a wide range of physiological processes that are crucial for healthy aging.

However, chronic stress can have a significant impact on sleep quality, leading to insomnia, fragmented sleep, and disrupted circadian rhythms. This, in turn, can exacerbate the negative effects of stress, creating a vicious cycle that can further accelerate the aging process.

By prioritizing sleep hygiene and adopting strategies to optimize their sleep quality, such as maintaining a consistent sleep schedule, creating a restful sleep environment, and practicing relaxation techniques before bed, individuals can better manage stress and support their overall longevity.

Integrating Stress Management into a Comprehensive Anti-Aging Lifestyle
As we have explored in this chapter, the management of stress and the cultivation of emotional well-being are essential components of a comprehensive anti-aging strategy. By addressing the profound impact that

stress can have on the aging process, individuals can unlock the full potential of their longevity journey and achieve a heightened sense of vitality and resilience.

However, it is important to recognize that stress management and emotional well-being do not exist in isolation; rather, they must be seamlessly integrated into a holistic approach to anti-aging that addresses other key aspects of health and lifestyle.

For example, the adoption of a nutrient-dense, anti-inflammatory diet can help mitigate the negative effects of stress by reducing oxidative stress and inflammation within the body. Similarly, regular physical activity not only benefits the cardiovascular and musculoskeletal systems but also promotes emotional well-being and stress resilience.

Furthermore, the optimization of sleep quality, as discussed earlier, can have a profound impact on an individual's ability to manage stress and maintain emotional equilibrium. By ensuring adequate, restorative sleep, individuals can better support their body's natural recovery processes and enhance their overall resilience to the challenges of aging.

Personalized Approach to Stress Management and Emotional Well-being

It is important to recognize that the path to stress management and emotional well-being is not a one-size-fits-all proposition. Each individual's response to stress and their unique emotional needs will vary, depending on factors such as their genetic predisposition, life experiences, and personal preferences.

By working closely with healthcare professionals, such as mental health therapists, counselors, or integrative medicine practitioners, individuals can develop a personalized stress management and emotional well-being plan that addresses their specific needs and challenges. This may involve a combination of techniques, including mindfulness-based practices, cognitive-behavioral therapy, biofeedback, and lifestyle interventions, all tailored to the individual's unique circumstances and goals.

Additionally, the integration of stress management and emotional well-being into an individual's anti-aging lifestyle may require ongoing adjustments and refinements as they navigate the dynamic landscape of aging. By remaining adaptable and open to exploring new strategies, individuals can ensure that their approach to stress and emotional health remains aligned with their evolving needs and priorities.

Embracing the Transformative Power of Emotional Well-being

As we embark on the journey of anti-aging, it is essential to recognize the profound and far-reaching impact that stress management and emotional well-being can have on our overall health and longevity. By cultivating a deep understanding of the mind-body connection and leveraging a comprehensive toolkit of stress-reducing techniques, individuals can not only mitigate the detrimental effects of chronic stress but also unlock the vast potential for vibrant, joyful, and fulfilling golden years.

Moreover, the pursuit of emotional well-being is not merely a means to an end; it is a transformative process that can enrich every aspect of an individual's life. By fostering positive emotions, nurturing meaningful relationships, and developing a resilient mindset, we can not only extend our lifespan but also enhance our "healthspan" – the period of our lives during which we thrive physically, mentally, and emotionally.

As you continue to navigate the complex landscape of anti-aging, remember that the path to longevity is not solely about optimizing physical health; it is also about cultivating a deep sense of inner peace, purpose, and connection. By embracing the power of stress management and emotional well-being, you can unlock the keys to a life that is not only longer but also richer, more vibrant, and more fulfilling.

CHAPTER 5

Sleep and Circadian Rhythms

In the quest for longevity and optimal health, the importance of quality sleep cannot be overstated. As we grow older, the age-related changes in our sleep patterns and circadian rhythms can have a profound impact on our overall well-being, contributing to a wide range of age-related conditions and accelerating the aging process.

In this chapter, we will explore the vital role that sleep and circadian rhythms play in the anti-aging equation, unveiling the science behind their impact on cellular function, metabolic health, and cognitive performance. By understanding the mechanisms that govern our sleep-wake cycles and adopting evidence-based strategies to optimize our sleep, we can unlock the secrets to a longer, healthier, and more vibrant life.

The Importance of Quality Sleep

Sleep, a fundamental physiological process that we all experience, is far more than just a period of rest and inactivity. During the various stages of sleep, our bodies and minds undergo a complex series of restorative and rejuvenating processes that are essential for maintaining optimal health and well-being.

However, as we age, the quality and quantity of our sleep can diminish, leading to a host of age-related challenges that can significantly impact our longevity and quality of life. Some of the key ways in which poor sleep can accelerate the aging process include:

1. Impaired Cellular Repair and Regeneration
   Sleep is a crucial period for cellular repair and regeneration, as it allows the body to divert resources towards the maintenance and rejuvenation of tissues and organs. During deep, slow-wave sleep, growth hormones are released, and cellular processes involved in DNA repair, protein synthesis, and tissue growth are upregulated.

As we grow older, the ability to achieve deep, restorative sleep can decline, leading to a diminished capacity for cellular rejuvenation. This, in turn, can contribute to the accumulation of DNA damage, the impairment of proteostasis (the balance of protein synthesis and degradation), and the accelerated deterioration of various bodily systems.

2. Metabolic Dysregulation and Increased Disease Risk
   Sleep plays a vital role in the regulation of our metabolic processes, including glucose homeostasis, hormone balance, and energy expenditure. Insufficient or poor-quality sleep has been linked to a range of age-related metabolic disorders, such as type 2 diabetes, obesity, and cardiovascular disease.

During sleep, the body's endocrine system undergoes important adjustments, with the release of hormones like insulin, leptin, and ghrelin being carefully synchronized. Disruptions to this delicate balance, as can occur with poor sleep, can lead to insulin resistance, increased inflammation, and a higher risk of developing metabolic diseases.

3. Cognitive Decline and Neurodegeneration
   The impact of sleep on cognitive function and brain health is particularly concerning in the context of aging. During sleep, the brain undergoes a series of essential processes, including the consolidation of memories, the clearance

of waste products, and the strengthening of neural connections.

Insufficient or fragmented sleep has been linked to a range of age-related cognitive impairments, such as decreased attention, impaired memory, and reduced problem-solving abilities. Moreover, poor sleep has been identified as a risk factor for the development of neurodegenerative diseases, like Alzheimer's and Parkinson's, by contributing to the accumulation of harmful proteins and the degeneration of brain cells.

4. Weakened Immune Function

Sleep plays a vital role in the proper functioning of the immune system, which can become increasingly compromised with age. During sleep, the body's immune cells are activated, and inflammatory markers are regulated, helping to maintain a balanced and resilient immune response.

However, chronic sleep disturbances can lead to the dysregulation of the immune system, contributing to the development of age-related immune disorders, an increased susceptibility to infections, and a diminished response to vaccinations – all of which can have a detrimental impact on longevity.

Optimizing Sleep for Cellular Rejuvenation

Given the profound impact that quality sleep can have on the aging process, the optimization of our sleep patterns and the alignment of our circadian rhythms should be a central component of any comprehensive anti-aging strategy.

Establishing Healthy Sleep Habits

One of the foundational steps in optimizing sleep for longevity is the adoption of healthy sleep habits. This includes:

1. Maintaining a consistent sleep schedule: Going to bed and waking up at

the same time, even on weekends, can help entrain the body's circadian rhythms.

2. Creating a sleep-conducive environment: Ensuring the bedroom is dark, cool, and quiet can promote better sleep quality.

3. Avoiding stimulants and screen time before bed: Caffeine, alcohol, and exposure to blue light-emitting devices can disrupt sleep.

4. Implementing relaxation techniques: Practices like meditation, deep breathing, or gentle yoga can help calm the mind and body before bed.

5. Avoiding daytime napping: While short power naps can be beneficial, prolonged daytime sleep can disrupt the sleep-wake cycle.

By consistently implementing these healthy sleep habits, individuals can lay the groundwork for improved sleep quality and support the body's natural rejuvenation processes.

Aligning Circadian Rhythms for Optimal Longevity

Closely tied to the importance of quality sleep is the alignment of our circadian rhythms – the internal 24-hour biological clock that governs a wide range of physiological and behavioral processes, including sleep-wake cycles, hormone secretion, and metabolic function.

As we age, the body's circadian rhythms can become increasingly disrupted, leading to a range of age-related issues, such as sleep disorders, cognitive impairment, and metabolic dysregulation. By understanding the mechanisms that govern these internal timekeepers and adopting strategies to optimize circadian alignment, individuals can unlock the full potential of sleep-related anti-aging benefits.

Some key strategies for aligning circadian rhythms include:

1. Exposure to natural light: Spending time outdoors during the day and

minimizing exposure to artificial light at night can help entrain the body's internal clock.

2. Maintaining a consistent sleep-wake schedule: Going to bed and waking up at the same time, even on weekends, can reinforce the body's circadian rhythms.
3. Engaging in regular physical activity: Exercise has been shown to enhance circadian alignment and improve sleep quality.
4. Avoiding disruptive behaviors: Minimizing exposure to blue light-emitting devices, consuming caffeine or alcohol late in the day, and altering sleep schedules can all disrupt circadian rhythms.
5. Considering light therapy or melatonin supplementation: In some cases, targeted interventions like light therapy or melatonin supplements may be beneficial for individuals struggling with circadian misalignment.

By prioritizing the alignment of their circadian rhythms and adopting evidence-based strategies to optimize their sleep, individuals can unlock a powerful synergy that supports cellular rejuvenation, metabolic health, and cognitive function – all of which are essential for the pursuit of longevity.

The Role of Sleep in Cellular Aging

At the cellular level, the impact of sleep on the aging process is particularly profound. During sleep, the body undergoes a series of essential restorative processes that are crucial for maintaining cellular health and longevity.

One of the key mechanisms by which sleep supports cellular rejuvenation is through the regulation of telomeres – the protective caps at the ends of our chromosomes. Telomere length is a crucial marker of cellular aging, as the gradual shortening of telomeres is associated with an increased risk of age-related diseases and overall mortality.

Interestingly, research has shown that sleep deprivation can accelerate telomere shortening, potentially contributing to the premature aging of cells.

Conversely, adequate, high-quality sleep has been linked to the maintenance of telomere length and the preservation of cellular integrity.

Furthermore, sleep plays a vital role in the clearing of cellular waste products and the repair of damaged DNA. During the various stages of sleep, the body's cellular cleanup and rejuvenation processes are upregulated, helping to remove harmful molecules, repair genetic material, and maintain the overall health of our cells.

This cellular-level impact of sleep is particularly relevant in the context of age-related diseases, such as neurodegenerative disorders and cancer. By supporting the body's ability to maintain healthy cells and prevent the accumulation of cellular damage, optimal sleep can help mitigate the risk of these age-related conditions and promote longevity.

Strategies for Improving Sleep Quality and Quantity

Given the profound importance of sleep in the anti-aging equation, it is essential to explore a range of evidence-based strategies that can help individuals improve the quality and quantity of their sleep.

Establishing a Robust Sleep Hygiene Routine

One of the foundational steps in optimizing sleep for longevity is the adoption of a comprehensive sleep hygiene routine. This can involve a combination of the following strategies:

1. Maintaining a consistent sleep-wake schedule: Going to bed and waking up at the same time, even on weekends, can help entrain the body's circadian rhythms.
2. Creating a sleep-conducive environment: Ensuring the bedroom is dark, cool, and quiet can promote better sleep quality.
3. Avoiding stimulants and screen time before bed: Caffeine, alcohol, and

exposure to blue light-emitting devices can disrupt sleep.

4. Implementing relaxation techniques: Practices like meditation, deep breathing, or gentle yoga can help calm the mind and body before bed.
5. Engaging in regular physical activity: Exercise has been shown to improve sleep quality, but it is important to avoid vigorous activity too close to bedtime.

By consistently implementing these sleep hygiene practices, individuals can lay the groundwork for improved sleep quality and support the body's natural rejuvenation processes.

Optimizing Circadian Alignment

As discussed earlier, the alignment of our circadian rhythms is crucial for maintaining optimal sleep and supporting longevity. By adopting strategies to optimize circadian alignment, individuals can further enhance the restorative benefits of sleep.

Some key strategies for aligning circadian rhythms include:

1. Exposure to natural light: Spending time outdoors during the day and minimizing exposure to artificial light at night can help entrain the body's internal clock.
2. Maintaining a consistent sleep-wake schedule: Going to bed and waking up at the same time, even on weekends, can reinforce the body's circadian rhythms.
3. Engaging in regular physical activity: Exercise has been shown to enhance circadian alignment and improve sleep quality.
4. Avoiding disruptive behaviors: Minimizing exposure to blue light-emitting devices, consuming caffeine or alcohol late in the day, and altering sleep schedules can all disrupt circadian rhythms.
5. Considering light therapy or melatonin supplementation: In some cases,

targeted interventions like light therapy or melatonin supplements may be beneficial for individuals struggling with circadian misalignment.

By prioritizing the alignment of their circadian rhythms and adopting evidence-based strategies to optimize their sleep, individuals can unlock a powerful synergy that supports cellular rejuvenation, metabolic health, and cognitive function – all of which are essential for the pursuit of longevity.

Personalized Approach to Sleep and Circadian Optimization

As with many aspects of the anti-aging journey, the path to optimal sleep and circadian alignment is not a one-size-fits-all proposition. Each individual's sleep and circadian needs can vary based on a range of factors, including age, genetic predisposition, lifestyle, and underlying health conditions.

By working closely with healthcare professionals, such as sleep specialists, integrative medicine practitioners, or chronobiologists, individuals can develop a personalized approach to sleep and circadian optimization. This may involve a combination of the strategies outlined in this chapter, as well as the incorporation of targeted interventions, such as sleep-focused cognitive-behavioral therapy, light therapy, or the use of customized supplements.

Furthermore, the optimization of sleep and circadian rhythms may require ongoing adjustments and refinements as individuals navigate the dynamic landscape of aging. By remaining adaptable and open to exploring new strategies, individuals can ensure that their approach to sleep and circadian alignment remains aligned with their evolving needs and priorities.

Embracing the Transformative Power of Sleep and Circadian Rhythms

As we have explored in this chapter, the optimization of sleep and the alignment of circadian rhythms are essential components of a comprehensive anti-aging strategy. By recognizing the profound impact that these physiological processes have on cellular health, metabolic function, and cognitive performance, individuals can unlock the keys to a longer, healthier, and more vibrant life.

Moreover, the pursuit of optimal sleep and circadian alignment is not merely a means to an end; it is a transformative process that can enrich every aspect of an individual's life. By cultivating a deep understanding of the body's internal timekeepers and implementing evidence-based strategies to support their natural rhythms, individuals can foster a heightened sense of vitality, resilience, and overall well-being.

As you continue your journey towards longevity, remember that the path to a longer, healthier life is not just about physical health – it is also about honoring the delicate balance of your body's natural processes. By embracing the power of sleep and circadian rhythms, you can unlock a world of cellular rejuvenation, metabolic optimization, and cognitive enhancement, empowering you to live your golden years with boundless energy, clarity, and joy.

So, let us embark on this sleep-centric odyssey together, recognizing that the key to unlocking the secrets of longevity lies not only in the hours we spend awake, but also in the precious time we devote to rest, restoration, and the alignment of our internal clocks. By prioritizing sleep and circadian health, we can pave the way for a future filled with vibrant, fulfilling, and well-rested days – a testament to the transformative power of this fundamental, yet often overlooked, aspect of the anti-aging journey.

CHAPTER 6

Hormone Balance and Regulation

As we age, our bodies undergo a complex series of hormonal changes that can have a profound impact on our overall health and longevity. The delicate balance of hormones, which play a crucial role in regulating a wide range of physiological processes, can become disrupted over time, leading to a host of age-related challenges that can accelerate the aging process.

In this chapter, we will explore the vital role that hormone balance and regulation play in the context of anti-aging, delving into the science behind the hormonal changes that accompany the aging process and uncovering the strategies that individuals can leverage to maintain hormonal equilibrium and support their longevity goals.

Understanding Age-Related Hormonal Changes

As we grow older, our bodies experience a gradual decline in the production and regulation of various hormones, including sex hormones, metabolic hormones, and stress hormones. These age-related hormonal changes can have far-reaching consequences on our physical and cognitive function, as well as our overall well-being.

Sex Hormones and Aging

One of the most well-known and impactful hormonal changes that occur with age is the decline in sex hormone production, particularly in the case of estrogen and testosterone.

In women, the onset of menopause is characterized by a significant reduction in estrogen levels, which can lead to a range of symptoms, such as hot flashes, mood changes, and vaginal atrophy. This hormonal shift has also been linked to an increased risk of age-related diseases, including osteoporosis, cardiovascular disease, and cognitive decline.

Similarly, men experience a gradual decline in testosterone production, a condition known as andropause or late-onset hypogonadism. This drop in testosterone levels can contribute to a loss of muscle mass, decreased libido, and impaired sexual function, as well as an increased risk of metabolic disorders and cardiovascular disease.

Metabolic Hormones and Aging
In addition to the changes in sex hormones, the aging process is also accompanied by alterations in the production and regulation of metabolic hormones, such as insulin, leptin, and thyroid hormones.

As we grow older, the body's sensitivity to insulin can diminish, leading to insulin resistance and an increased risk of type 2 diabetes. This metabolic dysregulation can have far-reaching consequences, including weight gain, cardiovascular disease, and cognitive impairment.

Similarly, the production of leptin, a hormone that regulates appetite and metabolism, can become disrupted with age, contributing to the age-related changes in body composition and energy balance. Thyroid hormones, which play a crucial role in regulating metabolism and energy expenditure, can also experience age-related fluctuations, further exacerbating metabolic challenges.

Stress Hormones and Aging

The aging process is also accompanied by changes in the body's stress response system, which is primarily regulated by the adrenal glands and the hypothalamic-pituitary-adrenal (HPA) axis.

As we grow older, the body's ability to mount an appropriate stress response can become impaired, leading to an imbalance in the production and regulation of stress hormones, such as cortisol. This chronic elevation of cortisol levels can have a detrimental impact on various aspects of health, including immune function, cognitive performance, and metabolic regulation.

These age-related hormonal changes, whether in the realm of sex hormones, metabolic hormones, or stress hormones, can have a profound and far-reaching impact on our overall health and longevity. By understanding the mechanisms behind these hormonal shifts and implementing targeted strategies to maintain hormonal equilibrium, individuals can unlock the secrets to a longer, healthier, and more vibrant life.

Strategies for Maintaining Hormonal Equilibrium

Given the pivotal role that hormone balance plays in the anti-aging equation, it is essential for individuals to explore a range of evidence-based strategies that can help them maintain hormonal equilibrium and support their longevity goals.

Optimizing Lifestyle Factors

One of the foundational approaches to maintaining hormonal balance is the optimization of various lifestyle factors, including diet, physical activity, and stress management.

Diet: The foods we consume can have a profound impact on the regulation and production of our hormones. By adopting a nutrient-dense, anti-inflammatory diet that is rich in whole, unprocessed foods, individuals can support hormonal balance and reduce the risk of age-related hormonal imbalances.

For example, incorporating healthy fats, such as those found in nuts, seeds, and avocados, can help support the production of sex hormones, while limiting the intake of refined carbohydrates and added sugars can improve insulin sensitivity and metabolic regulation.

Physical Activity: Regular physical activity has been shown to have a positive impact on hormonal balance, helping to maintain muscle mass, improve insulin sensitivity, and regulate the stress response.

Engaging in a well-rounded exercise regimen that includes both resistance training and cardiovascular exercise can help support the production and proper regulation of hormones like testosterone, growth hormone, and insulin.

Stress Management: As discussed in the previous chapter, chronic stress can have a detrimental impact on the body's stress response system, leading to an imbalance in the production and regulation of hormones like cortisol.

By incorporating stress-reducing techniques, such as mindfulness meditation, deep breathing exercises, or relaxation practices, individuals can help mitigate the negative effects of stress on their hormonal health and support overall longevity.

Targeted Supplementation
In addition to optimizing lifestyle factors, the strategic use of targeted supplements can also play a valuable role in maintaining hormonal equilibrium and supporting anti-aging efforts.

Some of the key supplements that have been explored for their potential to support hormonal balance include:

- Vitamin D: This essential nutrient has been shown to play a crucial role in the regulation of various hormones, including sex hormones and metabolic hormones.
- Omega-3 fatty acids: These healthy fats can help support the production and regulation of sex hormones, as well as reduce inflammation.
- Ashwagandha: This adaptogenic herb has been used in traditional medicine to help manage stress and support the body's stress response system.
- Saw Palmetto: This botanical supplement has been studied for its potential to help maintain healthy testosterone levels in men.
- Melatonin: This natural hormone, which regulates the sleep-wake cycle, has also been explored for its potential to support hormonal balance and longevity.

It is important to note that the use of any supplement should be done under the guidance of a healthcare professional, as the appropriate dosage and potential interactions can vary based on an individual's specific needs and health status.

Hormone Replacement Therapy

In some cases, individuals may require more targeted interventions, such as hormone replacement therapy (HRT), to address age-related hormonal imbalances and support their longevity goals.

HRT can involve the administration of synthetic or bioidentical hormones to help restore the body's hormonal equilibrium. This approach has been particularly well-studied in the context of menopausal and andropause-related hormonal changes, where the replacement of estrogen, progesterone, and/or testosterone can help alleviate symptoms and reduce the risk of age-related diseases.

However, the use of HRT is a complex and nuanced topic, as the potential benefits and risks can vary depending on factors such as the type of hormone, the delivery method, the timing of initiation, and the individual's overall health status.

Healthcare professionals, such as endocrinologists or integrative medicine practitioners, can work closely with individuals to assess their specific hormonal needs, weigh the potential risks and benefits, and develop a personalized HRT plan that aligns with their anti-aging goals and overall health priorities.

Personalized Approach to Hormonal Optimization

As with many aspects of the anti-aging journey, the path to maintaining hormonal equilibrium is not a one-size-fits-all proposition. Each individual's hormonal profile, genetic predispositions, and unique physiological characteristics can play a significant role in determining the most effective strategies for supporting their longevity goals.

By working closely with healthcare professionals, such as endocrinologists, integrative medicine practitioners, or functional medicine specialists, individuals can develop a personalized approach to hormonal optimization that addresses their specific needs and challenges.

This personalized approach may involve a combination of lifestyle interventions, targeted supplementation, and, in some cases, hormone replacement therapy. It may also require ongoing monitoring and adjustments as individuals navigate the dynamic landscape of aging and experience changes in their hormonal profiles.

Furthermore, the integration of hormonal optimization into a comprehensive anti-aging strategy is crucial, as the balance and regulation of hormones can have far-reaching implications for other aspects of health, such as metabolism, cognitive function, and immune function.

By embracing a personalized, holistic approach to hormonal equilibrium, individuals can unlock the full potential of their longevity journey, empowering them to live longer, healthier, and more vibrant lives.

The Role of Hormones in Longevity

As we have explored in this chapter, the delicate balance and regulation of hormones play a pivotal role in the anti-aging process, influencing a wide range of physiological and cognitive functions that are essential for maintaining optimal health and vitality.

Sex Hormones and Longevity

   The maintenance of healthy sex hormone levels, particularly in the case of estrogen and testosterone, has been linked to numerous anti-aging benefits.

In women, the preservation of estrogen levels can help maintain bone density, support cardiovascular health, and protect against cognitive decline. Similarly, in men, the maintenance of testosterone levels can help preserve muscle mass, improve sexual function, and reduce the risk of age-related metabolic disorders.

By implementing strategies to support the production and regulation of sex hormones, individuals can not only alleviate the symptoms associated with hormonal changes but also reduce their susceptibility to a wide range of age-related diseases, thereby enhancing their overall longevity.

Metabolic Hormones and Longevity

   The regulation of metabolic hormones, such as insulin, leptin, and thyroid hormones, is also crucial for supporting longevity and healthy aging.

Maintaining insulin sensitivity and optimal glucose metabolism can help prevent the development of type 2 diabetes, a condition that is closely linked to an increased risk of cardiovascular disease, cognitive impairment, and other age-related complications.

Similarly, the proper regulation of leptin and thyroid hormones can help support a healthy body composition, maintain energy balance, and optimize metabolic function – all of which are essential for promoting longevity and maintaining overall health and well-being.

Stress Hormones and Longevity

The body's stress response system, regulated primarily by the adrenal glands and the HPA axis, plays a critical role in the aging process. The proper regulation of stress hormones, such as cortisol, is essential for supporting immune function, cognitive performance, and overall resilience to the challenges of aging.

By implementing strategies to manage chronic stress and maintain a balanced stress response, individuals can help mitigate the detrimental effects of elevated cortisol levels, which have been linked to a wide range of age-related conditions, including inflammation, cognitive decline, and metabolic dysregulation.

Embracing the Transformative Power of Hormonal Equilibrium

As we embark on the quest for longevity, the pivotal role of hormone balance and regulation cannot be overstated. By understanding the complex interplay of sex hormones, metabolic hormones, and stress hormones, and by implementing targeted strategies to maintain hormonal equilibrium, individuals can unlock a world of anti-aging benefits that can profoundly impact their physical, mental, and emotional well-being.

Moreover, the pursuit of hormonal optimization is not merely a means to an end; it is a transformative process that can empower individuals to take control of their own aging trajectory and unlock the boundless potential of a longer, healthier, and more vibrant life.

By working closely with healthcare professionals and embracing a personalized approach to hormonal balance, individuals can create a synergistic effect that amplifies the benefits of their other anti-aging efforts, from optimizing nutrition and physical activity to cultivating emotional well-being and stress resilience.

As you continue your journey towards longevity, remember that the key to unlocking the secrets of a longer, healthier life lies not only in the external factors that we can control but also in the delicate internal mechanisms that govern our physiological processes. By prioritizing the maintenance of hormonal equilibrium, you can pave the way for a future filled with boundless energy, enhanced cognitive performance, and a heightened sense of overall well-being.

Embrace the transformative power of hormonal optimization, and embark on a path that not only extends the number of years you live but also enriches the quality of your golden days. Together, let us unlock the full potential of a life well-lived, one where the harmonious balance of our hormones serves as the foundation for a vibrant, rejuvenated, and enduring longevity.

CHAPTER 7

Brain Health and Cognitive Function

As we navigate the complexities of the aging process, the preservation of brain health and cognitive function emerges as a crucial priority. The mind, the very essence of our humanity, is not immune to the ravages of time, and the age-related decline in cognitive abilities can have a profound impact on our quality of life, independence, and overall well-being.

In this chapter, we will explore the intricate relationship between the aging brain and the pursuit of longevity, delving into the science behind age-related cognitive decline and uncovering the evidence-based strategies that individuals can leverage to maintain a sharp, resilient, and high-performing mind well into their golden years.

Understanding Age-Related Cognitive Decline

As we grow older, the brain, like other organs in the body, undergoes a series of structural and functional changes that can contribute to the gradual decline in cognitive abilities. This age-related cognitive decline, which can manifest in various forms, such as memory impairment, slowed processing speed, and reduced problem-solving skills, is a natural consequence of the aging process.

At the heart of this cognitive decline lies a complex interplay of cellular, molecular, and neurochemical changes that occur within the brain. Some of the key factors that contribute to the age-related deterioration of cognitive function include:

1. Neuronal Degeneration and Loss

One of the hallmarks of the aging brain is the gradual loss of neurons, the specialized cells that are responsible for information processing and communication within the central nervous system. Over time, the brain may experience neuronal degeneration, which can lead to a reduction in brain volume and a diminished capacity for cognitive function.

2. Synaptic Dysfunction and Altered Neurotransmitter Levels

The connections between neurons, known as synapses, play a crucial role in cognitive processes, such as learning and memory. As we age, the structure and function of these synapses can become compromised, leading to disruptions in the transmission of neural signals and the imbalance of important neurotransmitters, such as acetylcholine, dopamine, and serotonin.

3. Neuroinflammation and Oxidative Stress

Chronic inflammation and oxidative stress within the brain have been identified as key drivers of age-related cognitive decline. These processes can contribute to the damage and dysfunction of brain cells, impair synaptic plasticity, and disrupt the delicate balance of neurochemicals, ultimately leading to the deterioration of cognitive performance.

4. Vascular Changes and Cerebrovascular Damage

The aging process is also accompanied by changes in the brain's vascular system, including the narrowing of blood vessels and the impairment of blood flow. These vascular alterations can compromise the delivery of oxygen and nutrients to the brain, potentially contributing to the development of age-related cognitive impairments and increasing the risk of conditions like vascular dementia.

5. Accumulation of Harmful Proteins

The aging brain is also susceptible to the accumulation of harmful proteins, such as amyloid-beta and tau, which are hallmarks of neurodegenerative diseases like Alzheimer's. The buildup of these proteins can disrupt normal brain function, leading to the deterioration of cognitive abilities and the increased risk of dementia.

These age-related changes, which can occur in various combinations and degrees of severity, can have a significant impact on an individual's cognitive performance, ultimately affecting their ability to think, remember, and problem-solve effectively as they grow older.

Preventing Age-Related Cognitive Decline

Given the profound impact that age-related cognitive decline can have on an individual's quality of life and independence, the prevention and mitigation of these cognitive impairments should be a central focus of any comprehensive anti-aging strategy.

Fortunately, emerging research has shed light on a range of evidence-based interventions and lifestyle factors that can help support brain health and preserve cognitive function as we age.

Maintaining a Healthy Lifestyle

One of the foundational approaches to preventing age-related cognitive decline is the adoption of a healthy lifestyle that addresses multiple aspects of physical and mental well-being.

Nutrition: A nutrient-dense, anti-inflammatory diet that is rich in antioxidants, omega-3 fatty acids, and other brain-supporting nutrients can help protect the brain from the damaging effects of oxidative stress and inflammation.

Physical Activity: Regular physical exercise has been shown to have a positive impact on cognitive function, enhancing neuroplasticity, improving blood flow to the brain, and supporting the growth and maintenance of brain cells.

Stress Management: Chronic stress can have a detrimental effect on the brain, contributing to inflammation, neuronal damage, and the impairment of cognitive abilities. Incorporating stress-reducing techniques, such as mindfulness meditation, can help mitigate these negative impacts.

Sleep: As discussed in the previous chapter, maintaining optimal sleep quality and aligning circadian rhythms are crucial for supporting cognitive function and preventing age-related cognitive decline.

By seamlessly integrating these healthy lifestyle factors into their daily routines, individuals can create a powerful synergistic effect that promotes brain health and preserves cognitive abilities well into their later years.

Cognitive Training and Brain Stimulation
   In addition to the adoption of a healthy lifestyle, engaging in cognitive training and brain-stimulating activities can also play a significant role in maintaining and enhancing cognitive function as we age.

Cognitive Training: Activities that challenge the mind, such as puzzles, memory games, or learning a new skill, can help strengthen neural connections, improve cognitive flexibility, and support the brain's natural resilience to the aging process.

By regularly engaging in these types of cognitive exercises, individuals can not only maintain their current level of cognitive performance but also potentially enhance specific cognitive domains, such as memory, attention, or problem-solving skills.

Brain Stimulation: Emerging technologies and interventions, such as transcranial magnetic stimulation (TMS) or transcranial direct current stimulation (tDCS), have been explored for their potential to stimulate and enhance brain function.

These non-invasive brain stimulation techniques can help increase neuroplasticity, improve cognitive abilities, and potentially offset age-related cognitive decline. However, it is important to note that the long-term effects and safety of these interventions are still being studied, and they should be used under the guidance of healthcare professionals.

Targeted Nutritional Supplementation

While a nutrient-dense, whole-food-based diet should serve as the foundation for supporting brain health, the strategic use of targeted nutritional supplements can also play a valuable role in preserving cognitive function and preventing age-related cognitive decline.

Some of the key supplements that have been explored for their potential brain-boosting effects include:

- Omega-3 fatty acids: Found in fish oil or krill oil, these healthy fats have been linked to improved cognitive performance and a reduced risk of dementia.
- Antioxidants: Supplements containing vitamins C, E, and various polyphenols can help combat oxidative stress and support neuronal health.
- B vitamins: B vitamins, such as folate, B6, and B12, are essential for the proper functioning of the brain and the maintenance of cognitive abilities.
- Ginkgo biloba: This herbal supplement has been studied for its potential to improve blood flow to the brain and support cognitive function.
- Curcumin: The active compound in turmeric, curcumin has demonstrated anti-inflammatory and neuroprotective properties that may benefit the aging brain.

As with any supplement, it is crucial to consult with a healthcare professional to determine the appropriate dosage and to ensure that the use of these products aligns with an individual's unique health needs and goals.

Preventing Neurodegenerative Diseases

In the context of age-related cognitive decline, the prevention of neurodegenerative diseases, such as Alzheimer's and Parkinson's, is of particular importance. These debilitating conditions can have a profound impact on an individual's cognitive function, ultimately compromising their independence, quality of life, and overall well-being.

While the exact causes of neurodegenerative diseases are not yet fully understood, research has identified several risk factors and potential interventions that may help mitigate the development and progression of these conditions.

Lifestyle Factors: The adoption of a healthy lifestyle, as discussed earlier, can play a crucial role in reducing the risk of neurodegenerative diseases. Factors such as a nutrient-dense diet, regular physical activity, and stress management have all been associated with a lower incidence of these conditions.

Cognitive Stimulation: Engaging in cognitively stimulating activities, such as learning new skills, playing brain games, or pursuing intellectual hobbies, can help build cognitive reserve and potentially delay the onset of neurodegenerative diseases.

Targeted Interventions: In some cases, targeted interventions, such as the use of certain medications or the implementation of lifestyle modifications, may be explored under the guidance of healthcare professionals to address specific risk factors or underlying pathological processes associated with neurodegenerative diseases.

By proactively addressing the risk factors and leveraging the evidence-based strategies for supporting brain health, individuals can take a proactive approach to preventing the development of neurodegenerative diseases and preserving their cognitive function as they age.

Personalized Approaches to Brain Health and Cognitive Function

As with many aspects of the anti-aging journey, the path to maintaining and enhancing cognitive function is not a one-size-fits-all proposition. Each individual's brain health and cognitive abilities are influenced by a unique combination of genetic, environmental, and lifestyle factors, necessitating a personalized approach to optimization.

By working closely with healthcare professionals, such as neurologists, neuropsychologists, or integrative medicine practitioners, individuals can develop a tailored plan that addresses their specific needs and challenges. This personalized approach may involve a combination of the strategies outlined in this chapter, as well as the incorporation of targeted interventions based on an individual's genetic profile, cognitive assessments, and overall health status.

For example, some individuals may benefit more from a specific type of cognitive training program, while others may require a more comprehensive approach that addresses underlying health conditions, such as metabolic disorders or cardiovascular health. Similarly, the use of targeted nutritional supplements or brain stimulation techniques may be more appropriate for some individuals based on their unique neurochemical profiles and cognitive strengths and weaknesses.

Furthermore, the integration of brain health and cognitive function optimization into a broader anti-aging strategy is crucial, as the health and performance of the brain are inextricably linked to various other physiological and psychological processes. By adopting a holistic approach that addresses factors such as physical activity, stress management, and hormonal balance, individuals can create a synergistic effect that enhances the resilience and longevity of their cognitive abilities.

Embracing the Transformative Power of Brain Health

As we embark on the journey of anti-aging, the preservation of brain health and cognitive function emerges as a critical priority, as the mind is the very essence of our humanity and the key to our independence, productivity, and overall well-being.

By embracing the strategies and interventions outlined in this chapter, individuals can unlock the transformative power of a sharp, resilient, and high-performing brain, empowering them to navigate the challenges of aging with clarity, adaptability, and a profound sense of purpose.

Moreover, the pursuit of brain health is not merely a means to an end; it is a transformative process that can enrich every aspect of an individual's life. By cultivating a deep understanding of the aging brain and actively engaging in activities that support cognitive function, individuals can foster a heightened sense of mental agility, emotional resilience, and overall well-being.

As you continue your journey towards longevity, remember that the key to unlocking the secrets of a longer, healthier life lies not only in the optimization of your physical health but also in the nourishment and preservation of your most essential asset – your mind. By prioritizing brain health and cognitive function, you can pave the way for a future filled with mental clarity, problem-solving prowess, and the ability to fully engage with the world around you.

Embrace the transformative power of brain health, and embark on a path that not only extends the number of years you live but also enriches the quality of your golden days. Together, let us unlock the full potential of a life well-lived, where the vitality and resilience of our minds serve as the foundation for a vibrant, rejuvenated, and enduring longevity.

CHAPTER 8

Skin and Beauty Maintenance

As we navigate the complexities of the aging process, the health and appearance of our skin emerges as a crucial concern. The skin, our largest organ, serves as a visible reflection of our overall well-being, and the age-related changes that occur within this dynamic system can have a profound impact on our self-perception, confidence, and quality of life.

In this chapter, we will delve into the science behind skin aging, exploring the various intrinsic and extrinsic factors that contribute to the deterioration of skin health and appearance. Furthermore, we will uncover a comprehensive range of evidence-based strategies and interventions that individuals can leverage to protect, nourish, and rejuvenate their skin, empowering them to maintain a vibrant, youthful, and radiant complexion well into their golden years.

Understanding the Aging of Skin

The process of skin aging is a complex, multifaceted phenomenon that is influenced by a combination of intrinsic and extrinsic factors. Understanding the underlying mechanisms that drive skin aging is essential for the development of effective anti-aging strategies and the maintenance of optimal skin health.

Intrinsic Skin Aging

Intrinsic skin aging, also known as chronological aging, refers to the natural, genetically-programmed changes that occur within the skin over time. These age-related changes are primarily driven by the gradual deterioration of cellular and molecular processes, leading to the following manifestations:

1. Decreased Cellular Turnover: As we grow older, the rate of skin cell renewal and proliferation slows down, resulting in a thinner, more fragile epidermis (the outermost layer of skin).

2. Reduced Collagen and Elastin Production: The skin's structural proteins, collagen, and elastin, responsible for maintaining firmness and elasticity, decline in production and quality, leading to the development of wrinkles and sagging.

3. Diminished Hyaluronic Acid Levels: Hyaluronic acid, a crucial component of the skin's extracellular matrix, decreases with age, contributing to the loss of skin moisture and volume.

4. Impaired Barrier Function: The skin's natural barrier, which protects against environmental stressors and maintains hydration, becomes less effective, leading to increased transepidermal water loss and vulnerability to external insults.

5. Compromised Vascular and Lymphatic Systems: The aging process can impair the skin's blood and lymphatic vessels, reducing nutrient and oxygen supply, as well as waste removal, which can lead to a dull, uneven complexion.

Extrinsic Skin Aging

In addition to the intrinsic, genetically-driven changes, the skin is also susceptible to various extrinsic, or environmental, factors that can accelerate the aging process. These include:

1. UV Exposure: Ultraviolet (UV) radiation from the sun is a primary driver of extrinsic skin aging, contributing to the development of wrinkles, age spots, and an increased risk of skin cancer.

2. Pollution and Environmental Stressors: Exposure to air pollutants, cigarette smoke, and other environmental toxins can generate free radicals and induce oxidative stress, leading to premature aging of the skin.

3. Unhealthy Lifestyle Habits: Factors such as poor diet, lack of exercise, chronic stress, and insufficient sleep can all negatively impact the skin's health and appearance.

4. Repetitive Facial Expressions: Frequent and intense facial expressions, such as squinting or frowning, can contribute to the formation of dynamic wrinkles over time.

The interplay between intrinsic and extrinsic factors, combined with individual genetic predispositions, create a complex and dynamic landscape of skin aging, necessitating a comprehensive approach to maintaining optimal skin health and appearance.

Protecting Skin from Environmental Stressors

Recognizing the significant role that environmental factors play in the aging of the skin, the implementation of effective strategies to protect the skin from external stressors becomes a crucial component of any anti-aging regimen.

Sun Protection

As the primary driver of extrinsic skin aging, UV radiation from the sun is a formidable foe that must be addressed with diligence and consistency. Comprehensive sun protection is essential for preventing premature wrinkles, age spots, and an increased risk of skin cancer.

Key sun protection strategies include:

1. Applying broad-spectrum sunscreen with an SPF of 30 or higher, and reapplying it every 2 hours during sun exposure.
2. Seeking shade and avoiding direct sun exposure, especially during peak UV hours (10 AM to 4 PM).
3. Wearing protective clothing, such as wide-brimmed hats, long-sleeved shirts, and UV-blocking sunglasses.

By making sun protection a daily habit, individuals can significantly mitigate the damaging effects of UV radiation and preserve the health and youthful appearance of their skin.

Pollution and Environmental Protection

In addition to sun exposure, the skin is also vulnerable to the harmful effects of air pollution, cigarette smoke, and other environmental toxins. These environmental stressors can generate free radicals, induce oxidative stress, and disrupt the skin's natural barrier function, leading to premature aging and a compromised complexion.

To protect the skin from these environmental insults, individuals can consider the following strategies:

1. Using antioxidant-rich skincare products, such as those containing vitamins C and E, to neutralize free radicals and support the skin's natural defenses.
2. Incorporating air purifiers or investing in high-quality air filtration systems to reduce exposure to airborne pollutants.
3. Avoiding exposure to cigarette smoke and other known environmental toxins whenever possible.

4. Maintaining a healthy lifestyle, including a nutrient-dense diet and regular exercise, to strengthen the skin's resilience.

By proactively addressing both UV exposure and environmental stressors, individuals can create a comprehensive shield to safeguard the health and appearance of their skin.

Topical Treatments and Cosmetic Procedures

While protective measures are essential for preventing further skin damage, individuals can also explore a range of topical treatments and cosmetic procedures to address existing age-related concerns and promote skin rejuvenation.

Topical Skincare Formulations

Advances in the field of dermatology and cosmetic science have led to the development of a wide array of topical skincare products designed to target specific signs of aging and support overall skin health.

Some of the key active ingredients and formulations that have demonstrated anti-aging benefits include:

1. Retinoids: Derivatives of vitamin A, such as retinol and tretinoin, can stimulate collagen production, improve skin texture, and minimize the appearance of fine lines and wrinkles.
2. Alpha-Hydroxy Acids (AHAs): Compounds like glycolic acid and lactic acid can gently exfoliate the skin, promote cell turnover, and improve hydration.
3. Antioxidants: Vitamins C and E, as well as coenzyme Q10 and resveratrol, can help neutralize free radicals and protect the skin from environmental damage.

4. Peptides: These short chains of amino acids can signal the skin to produce more collagen, elastin, and hyaluronic acid, leading to firmer, more youthful-looking skin.
5. Growth Factors: Topical serums containing growth factors, such as epidermal growth factor (EGF) and fibroblast growth factor (FGF), can stimulate cellular repair and rejuvenation.

When incorporating these topical treatments into a skincare regimen, it is essential to work closely with a dermatologist or skincare professional to ensure the products are appropriate for an individual's skin type and concerns, and to avoid potential irritation or adverse reactions.

Cosmetic Procedures

In addition to topical skincare, individuals may also choose to explore various cosmetic procedures to address more advanced signs of skin aging and achieve a more youthful, radiant appearance.

Some of the most common anti-aging cosmetic procedures include:

1. Injectables: Botulinum toxin (Botox) and dermal fillers can temporarily smooth out dynamic wrinkles, restore volume, and improve the overall appearance of the skin.
2. Laser Treatments: Ablative and non-ablative laser therapies can stimulate collagen production, improve skin texture, and minimize the appearance of age spots and sun damage.
3. Chemical Peels: Varying concentrations of alpha-hydroxy acids or trichloroacetic acid can exfoliate the skin, reduce the visibility of fine lines and discoloration, and promote a more youthful, radiant complexion.
4. Microneedling: This minimally invasive procedure uses fine needles to create micro-injuries in the skin, triggering the body's natural healing

response and stimulating the production of collagen and elastin.

5. Radiofrequency (RF) Treatments: RF energy can be used to tighten and lift sagging skin, improve skin texture, and reduce the appearance of wrinkles.

It is crucial to consult with a licensed and experienced dermatologist or plastic surgeon when considering any cosmetic procedures, as they can provide personalized guidance, assess an individual's suitability, and develop a comprehensive treatment plan that aligns with their specific skin concerns and goals.

Lifestyle Factors for Youthful Skin

While topical treatments and cosmetic procedures can certainly play a role in maintaining a vibrant, youthful complexion, the foundation for healthy, age-resistant skin lies in the adoption of a comprehensive, lifestyle-based approach.

Nutrition and Hydration

The foods we consume and the fluids we ingest can have a profound impact on the health and appearance of our skin. By prioritizing a nutrient-dense, anti-inflammatory diet rich in antioxidants, healthy fats, and hydrating compounds, individuals can support the skin's natural rejuvenation processes and minimize the visible signs of aging.

Some key dietary considerations for youthful skin include:

- Incorporating omega-3-rich foods, such as fatty fish, chia seeds, and walnuts, to reduce inflammation and support the skin's barrier function.
- Eating a variety of brightly colored fruits and vegetables, which are abundant in skin-nourishing vitamins, minerals, and antioxidants.
- Staying hydrated by drinking plenty of water and consuming water-rich

foods like cucumbers, watermelon, and leafy greens.

- Limiting the intake of processed, sugar-laden foods, which can contribute to oxidative stress and premature aging of the skin.

Physical Activity and Stress Management

In addition to a healthy diet, regular physical activity and effective stress management techniques can also play a crucial role in maintaining the health and appearance of the skin.

Exercise has been shown to improve blood circulation, enhance the delivery of nutrients to the skin, and support the skin's natural detoxification processes. Furthermore, the reduction of stress and the promotion of overall well-being can help mitigate the detrimental effects of chronic inflammation and oxidative stress on the skin.

Incorporating a range of physical activities, such as aerobic exercise, strength training, and mind-body practices like yoga or Tai Chi, can help individuals achieve a holistic approach to skin health and rejuvenation. Additionally, the implementation of stress-reducing techniques, such as meditation, deep breathing, or guided imagery, can further support the skin's resilience and vitality.

Sleep and Skin Health

The importance of quality sleep in the context of skin health and appearance cannot be overstated. During the various stages of sleep, the body undergoes a series of restorative and rejuvenating processes that are essential for maintaining the health and youthfulness of the skin.

Adequate, high-quality sleep has been shown to support the skin's natural barrier function, enhance collagen production, and promote the clearance of toxins and waste products from the skin. Conversely, chronic sleep deprivation can lead to increased inflammation, impaired skin barrier function, and a dull, tired-looking complexion.

By prioritizing consistent, restorative sleep and aligning their circadian rhythms, individuals can create an optimal environment for the skin's natural rejuvenation processes, ultimately supporting a more vibrant, youthful, and radiant complexion.

Personalized Skin Health and Beauty Maintenance

As with many aspects of the anti-aging journey, the path to maintaining optimal skin health and appearance is not a one-size-fits-all proposition. Each individual's skin type, genetic predispositions, and unique environmental exposures can influence the most effective strategies for achieving a youthful, radiant complexion.

By working closely with skincare professionals, such as dermatologists, estheticians, or integrative medicine practitioners, individuals can develop a personalized skin health and beauty maintenance plan that addresses their specific needs and concerns. This personalized approach may involve a combination of the strategies outlined in this chapter, as well as the incorporation of targeted treatments, customized skincare regimens, and lifestyle modifications tailored to the individual's unique skin characteristics and goals.

For example, some individuals may require a more robust sun protection regimen due to their skin's sensitivity to UV radiation, while others may benefit more from the incorporation of specific active ingredients, such as retinoids or growth factors, based on their skin's responsiveness and underlying concerns.

Furthermore, the integration of skin health and beauty maintenance into a broader anti-aging strategy is crucial, as the health and appearance of the skin are inextricably linked to various other physiological and psychological processes. By adopting a holistic approach that addresses factors such as nutrition, stress management, and hormone balance, individuals can create a synergistic effect that enhances the resilience and youthfulness of their skin.

Embracing the Transformative Power of Skin Health and Beauty

As we navigate the complexities of the aging process, the maintenance of skin health and beauty emerges as a vital component of a comprehensive anti-aging strategy. By recognizing the profound impact that the skin's appearance can have on our self-confidence, overall well-being, and quality of life, individuals can unlock the transformative power of a vibrant, youthful, and radiant complexion.

Moreover, the pursuit of skin health and beauty is not merely a superficial endeavor; it is a transformative process that can enrich every aspect of an individual's life. By cultivating a deep understanding of the skin's intricate biology and actively engaging in practices that support its health and rejuvenation, individuals can foster a heightened sense of self-esteem, confidence, and overall well-being.

As you continue your journey towards longevity, remember that the key to unlocking the secrets of a longer, healthier life lies not only in the optimization of your internal physiological processes but also in the nourishment and protection of your skin – the very canvas upon which your life's story is written.

By prioritizing skin health and beauty maintenance, you can pave the way for a future filled with radiant, youthful skin that reflects the vitality and resilience of your entire being. Embrace the transformative power of skin health, and embark on a path that not only extends the number of years you live but also enriches the quality of your golden days.

Together, let us unlock the full potential of a life well-lived, where the vibrancy and resilience of our skin serve as the foundation for a holistic, rejuvenated, and enduring longevity.

CHAPTER 9

Genetic and Epigenetic Factors in Aging

As we delve deeper into the complexities of the aging process, the role of genetics and epigenetics emerges as a crucial area of exploration. The human genome, with its intricate tapestry of genetic instructions, plays a pivotal part in shaping the trajectory of our longevity, while epigenetic modifications – the dynamic and reversible changes that influence gene expression without altering the underlying DNA sequence – can further modulate the pace and expression of the aging phenotype.

In this chapter, we will delve into the fascinating world of genomics and epigenetics, uncovering the latest scientific discoveries and their implications for the pursuit of longevity. By understanding the genetic underpinnings of aging and the ways in which epigenetic factors can be leveraged to promote healthy longevity, individuals can unlock the secrets to a longer, healthier, and more vibrant life.

Exploring the Genomics of Longevity

The field of genomics, which encompasses the study of the human genome and its role in various biological processes, has provided invaluable insights into the genetic basis of aging and longevity. By identifying specific genetic variants and their associated effects, researchers have been able to shed light on the complex interplay between an individual's genetic makeup and their susceptibility to age-related diseases and overall lifespan.

Genetic Determinants of Longevity

One of the primary areas of focus in the genomics of longevity is the identification of genetic variants that are associated with exceptional longevity, or the ability to reach advanced ages while maintaining good health and cognitive function.

Through large-scale genome-wide association studies (GWAS) and the analysis of centenarian populations, researchers have uncovered a number of genetic loci and specific gene variants that are more commonly found in individuals who have achieved exceptional longevity. Some of the key genes and pathways that have been linked to longevity include:

1. Sirtuins (SIRT1-SIRT7): This family of genes plays a crucial role in regulating cellular processes, such as DNA repair, mitochondrial function, and metabolic homeostasis, all of which are important for healthy aging.

2. Insulin/IGF-1 Signaling Pathway: Genetic variants that are associated with decreased insulin/IGF-1 signaling have been linked to extended lifespan in various model organisms, as well as in some human populations.

3. APOE Gene: The APOE gene, which is involved in cholesterol metabolism, has been extensively studied in the context of longevity and age-related diseases, such as Alzheimer's disease.

4. Telomere-Related Genes: Genes that influence telomere length and maintenance, such as TERT and TERC, have been associated with exceptional longevity and a reduced risk of age-related diseases.

By understanding the genetic underpinnings of longevity, researchers can begin to develop personalized strategies for promoting healthy aging, based on an individual's unique genetic profile and the targeted modulation of key longevity-associated pathways.

Genetic Predisposition to Age-Related Diseases

In addition to the identification of longevity-associated genes, genomic research has also shed light on the genetic factors that may predispose individuals to various age-related diseases, such as cardiovascular disease, cancer, and neurodegenerative disorders.

By examining the genetic variants and gene-environment interactions that contribute to the development and progression of these age-related conditions, researchers can help individuals better understand their personal risk profiles and tailor their preventive and management strategies accordingly.

For example, the identification of specific genetic markers associated with an increased risk of Alzheimer's disease can allow individuals to take proactive steps to maintain cognitive function, such as engaging in regular physical and mental exercise, optimizing their sleep and stress management, and potentially exploring targeted interventions or therapies.

Similarly, genetic insights into the predisposition to cardiovascular diseases can empower individuals to adopt lifestyle modifications, such as a heart-healthy diet, regular physical activity, and the management of risk factors like hypertension and diabetes, to mitigate their genetic susceptibility.

By leveraging the power of genomics, individuals can take a more personalized and proactive approach to their health and longevity, tailoring their preventive strategies and interventions to address their unique genetic predispositions and maximize their chances of achieving a longer, healthier life.

Epigenetic Modifications and Anti-Aging Strategies

While the study of genomics has provided invaluable insights into the genetic basis of aging and longevity, the field of epigenetics has emerged as an equally pivotal area of exploration. Epigenetics refers to the dynamic and reversible changes in gene expression that occur without alterations to the underlying DNA sequence, and these modifications can have a profound impact on the aging process and the development of age-related diseases.

The Epigenetic Hallmarks of Aging

As we grow older, our cells and tissues undergo a series of epigenetic changes that contribute to the aging phenotype. These epigenetic hallmarks of aging include:

1. DNA Methylation Changes: The addition or removal of methyl groups to specific regions of the DNA can lead to the silencing or activation of certain genes, influencing cellular function and the aging trajectory.

2. Histone Modifications: Changes in the chemical modifications of histone proteins, which package and organize DNA within the cell, can alter gene expression patterns and contribute to the aging process.

3. Chromatin Remodeling: The reorganization of chromatin, the complex of DNA and proteins that make up the genetic material, can impact the accessibility of genetic information and the regulation of age-related genes.

4. Non-Coding RNA Dysregulation: The imbalance or altered expression of non-coding RNAs, such as microRNAs and long non-coding RNAs, can disrupt crucial cellular processes and contribute to the development of age-related diseases.

5. Cellular Senescence: The accumulation of senescent cells, which have permanently ceased division, can lead to the release of inflammatory factors and the promotion of age-related pathologies.

Understanding the epigenetic hallmarks of aging is crucial, as it allows researchers and healthcare professionals to identify potential targets for intervention and the development of strategies aimed at promoting healthy longevity.

Epigenetic Interventions for Anti-Aging

Given the dynamic and reversible nature of epigenetic modifications, the field of anti-aging has increasingly focused on the development of interventions that can favorably modulate the epigenetic landscape and support healthy aging.

Some of the key epigenetic interventions being explored for their anti-aging potential include:

1. Dietary and Nutritional Approaches: Certain bioactive compounds found in foods, such as folate, vitamin B12, and polyphenols, have been shown to influence epigenetic mechanisms and support healthy aging.

2. Physical Activity and Exercise: Regular physical activity can trigger epigenetic changes that enhance mitochondrial function, reduce inflammation, and promote the maintenance of cellular health and longevity.

3. Stress Management Techniques: Practices like mindfulness meditation and yoga have been associated with epigenetic modifications that can mitigate the harmful effects of chronic stress on the aging process.

4. Pharmacological Interventions: Medications and compounds that target specific epigenetic regulators, such as histone deacetylase (HDAC) inhibitors and DNA methyltransferase (DNMT) inhibitors, are being investigated for their potential to delay or reverse age-related diseases.

5. Calorie Restriction and Fasting Mimetics: Dietary interventions that mimic the effects of calorie restriction, such as intermittent fasting, have been found to induce epigenetic changes that can promote longevity and

healthspan.

By leveraging these epigenetic interventions and tailoring them to an individual's unique genetic and environmental factors, healthcare professionals can help create personalized anti-aging strategies that address the dynamic and multifaceted nature of the aging process.

Personalized Approaches to Genetic and Epigenetic Optimization

As the fields of genomics and epigenetics continue to evolve, the importance of adopting a personalized approach to anti-aging interventions becomes increasingly evident. Each individual's genetic makeup and epigenetic profile are unique, necessitating a tailored strategy that addresses their specific needs and vulnerabilities.

Genetic Testing and Risk Assessment

One of the key components of a personalized approach to anti-aging is the utilization of genetic testing and risk assessment tools. By analyzing an individual's genetic profile, healthcare professionals can identify specific genetic variants and risk factors that may influence their susceptibility to age-related diseases and guide the development of targeted preventive strategies.

Genetic testing panels, such as those that assess the risk of Alzheimer's disease, cardiovascular disease, or certain types of cancer, can provide valuable insights into an individual's genetic predispositions. Armed with this information, individuals can then work with their healthcare team to implement a comprehensive plan that addresses their specific genetic vulnerabilities, which may include lifestyle modifications, targeted screening and monitoring, or the exploration of preventive interventions.

Epigenetic Profiling and Optimization

In addition to genetic testing, the assessment and optimization of an individual's epigenetic profile can also play a crucial role in the personalization of anti-aging strategies. By analyzing the epigenetic markers associated with the aging process, healthcare professionals can identify areas of concern and develop targeted interventions to favorably modulate the epigenetic landscape.

This may involve the implementation of lifestyle-based approaches, such as dietary modifications, physical activity regimens, and stress management techniques, all of which have been shown to influence epigenetic mechanisms and support healthy longevity. In some cases, the use of pharmacological or nutraceutical interventions that target specific epigenetic regulators may also be considered, but this should be done under the close supervision of a healthcare provider.

The integration of genetic and epigenetic information, in combination with an individual's overall health status, environmental factors, and personal preferences, allows for the creation of a truly personalized anti-aging plan that addresses the multifaceted nature of the aging process.

Harnessing the Power of Personalized Genomics and Epigenetics

As we continue to unravel the complex interplay between genetics, epigenetics, and the aging process, the potential for personalized anti-aging strategies to transform the landscape of longevity becomes increasingly apparent.

By leveraging the insights gleaned from genomic and epigenetic research, individuals can take a proactive and targeted approach to maintaining their health and vitality well into their golden years. This may involve the implementation of lifestyle modifications that address their specific genetic predispositions, the exploration of preventive interventions tailored to their epigenetic profile, or the incorporation of emerging therapies that directly target the molecular underpinnings of the aging process.

Moreover, the pursuit of personalized anti-aging strategies extends beyond just the physical aspects of health and longevity. By understanding the genetic and epigenetic factors that shape an individual's susceptibility to age-related cognitive decline, mental health challenges, or even the preservation of physical appearance, healthcare professionals can help individuals create a comprehensive plan that addresses the multidimensional nature of the aging experience.

As you continue your journey towards longevity, remember that the key to unlocking the secrets of a longer, healthier life lies not only in the adoption of broad, one-size-fits-all interventions but also in the tailored and personalized approach that considers the unique characteristics of your genetic and epigenetic profile. By embracing the power of personalized genomics and epigenetics, you can pave the way for a future filled with optimal health, enhanced resilience, and the boundless potential of a life well-lived.

Embark on this transformative path, where the insights gleaned from the human genome and the dynamic epigenetic landscape serve as the foundation for a comprehensive, individualized anti-aging strategy. Together, let us unlock the full potential of a longevity journey that is as unique as the individuals who embark upon it, truly embracing the promise of a vibrant, rejuvenated, and enduring future.

CHAPTER 10

Supplementation and Nutraceuticals

As we delve deeper into the pursuit of longevity, the strategic use of dietary supplements and nutraceuticals has emerged as a powerful tool in the anti-aging arsenal. While a nutrient-dense, whole-food-based diet should serve as the foundation of any comprehensive longevity strategy, the incorporation of targeted supplements and bioactive compounds can provide an additional layer of support, addressing specific nutritional gaps and leveraging the latest scientific advancements in the field of healthy aging.

In this chapter, we will explore the role of dietary supplements and nutraceuticals in the context of anti-aging, uncovering the latest research on their potential benefits, as well as the importance of safety and personalization when incorporating these products into one's longevity regimen.

The Role of Dietary Supplements in Anti-Aging

Dietary supplements, which can encompass a wide range of vitamins, minerals, herbs, and other bioactive compounds, can play a valuable role in supporting the body's natural defenses against the ravages of time. By targeting specific physiological processes and addressing nutritional deficiencies, these supplements can help bolster cellular health, mitigate age-related decline, and promote overall longevity.

Vitamins and Minerals for Longevity

Certain vitamins and minerals have been extensively studied for their potential to support healthy aging and combat the effects of the aging process.

Vitamin C: A potent antioxidant, vitamin C has been linked to the reduction of oxidative stress, the enhancement of immune function, and the support of collagen production – all of which are crucial for maintaining skin health and overall tissue integrity.

Vitamin E: This fat-soluble antioxidant can help protect cellular membranes from the damaging effects of free radicals, potentially reducing the risk of age-related diseases, such as cardiovascular disease and cognitive decline.

Vitamin D: Beyond its well-known role in bone health, vitamin D has also been associated with the modulation of inflammatory pathways, the enhancement of immune function, and the support of cognitive performance – all of which are essential for healthy aging.

Zinc: This essential mineral plays a vital role in the proper functioning of the immune system, the maintenance of cellular integrity, and the regulation of gene expression – factors that are crucial for longevity.

Magnesium: As a cofactor for numerous enzymatic reactions, magnesium is essential for energy production, muscle and nerve function, and the regulation of blood pressure – all of which can decline with age.

By ensuring an adequate intake of these and other key vitamins and minerals, individuals can help support a wide range of physiological processes that are integral to the anti-aging equation.

Omega-3 Fatty Acids: The Anti-Inflammatory Champions

Omega-3 fatty acids, such as those found in fish oil or krill oil, have long been recognized for their potent anti-inflammatory properties, which are essential for maintaining overall health and combating the age-related increase in chronic inflammation.

Numerous studies have linked the supplementation of omega-3 fatty acids to a reduced risk of cardiovascular disease, cognitive decline, and certain types of cancer – all of which are common age-related conditions. These healthy fats can also support the maintenance of telomere length, a crucial marker of cellular aging, and promote the health and function of the immune system.

By incorporating omega-3 supplements into their longevity regimen, individuals can help counteract the damaging effects of inflammation and support the body's natural resilience to the challenges of aging.

Antioxidant Supplements: Neutralizing Free Radicals

The accumulation of oxidative stress and free radical damage is a hallmark of the aging process, contributing to the deterioration of cellular function and the development of various age-related diseases. Antioxidant supplements can play a vital role in mitigating these harmful effects and promoting cellular health.

Some of the key antioxidant supplements with potential anti-aging benefits include:

- Coenzyme Q10 (CoQ10): This essential cofactor for energy production has been linked to the protection of mitochondrial function and the reduction of cardiovascular disease risk.

- Resveratrol: This polyphenol compound, found in red wine and certain berries, has been studied for its ability to activate longevity-associated pathways and support healthy aging.

- Curcumin: The active compound in turmeric, curcumin, has demonstrated potent anti-inflammatory and neuroprotective properties that may benefit the aging brain.

- Glutathione: This endogenous antioxidant plays a crucial role in the body's detoxification processes and can help neutralize free radicals and support cellular health.

By incorporating a variety of antioxidant supplements into their daily routine, individuals can help strengthen their body's natural defenses against the ravages of oxidative stress and promote overall cellular resilience.

Evidence-Based Supplements for Longevity

While the benefits of vitamins, minerals, and antioxidants in the context of anti-aging are well-established, the field of dietary supplementation continues to evolve, with researchers exploring a range of other bioactive compounds and their potential to support healthy longevity.

Adaptogens: Promoting Stress Resilience

Adaptogens are a class of natural herbs and botanicals that have been shown to help the body adapt to and overcome the negative effects of stress. As chronic stress is a major contributor to the aging process, the incorporation of adaptogenic supplements can play a crucial role in supporting overall resilience and well-being.

Some of the most well-studied adaptogens with potential anti-aging benefits include:

- Ashwagandha: This Ayurvedic herb has been linked to the reduction of cortisol levels, the enhancement of cognitive function, and the support of immune health.
   - Rhodiola: This arctic root has been associated with improved physical and mental endurance, as well as the modulation of stress-related pathways.
   - Ginseng: Both Asian and American ginseng have been explored for their ability to combat fatigue, support mood, and potentially enhance longevity.

By helping the body better adapt to and recover from the physiological and psychological stresses of daily life, adaptogens can contribute to the maintenance of overall health and the promotion of healthy aging.

Telomere-Supportive Supplements

As discussed in previous chapters, the length and integrity of telomeres, the protective caps at the ends of our chromosomes, are closely linked to cellular aging and overall longevity. Accordingly, supplements that support telomere health have become a focus of anti-aging research.

Certain nutrients and compounds, such as vitamin C, vitamin E, omega-3 fatty acids, and the amino acid N-acetylcysteine, have been associated with the maintenance of telomere length and the reduction of telomere attrition. Additionally, the supplementation of specific plant-derived compounds, like astaxanthin and pterostilbene, has also been explored for their potential to support telomere health and promote cellular longevity.

By incorporating telomere-supportive supplements into their longevity regimen, individuals can help protect the integrity of their genetic material and potentially slow down the pace of cellular aging.

Gut Health and Longevity Supplements

The gut microbiome, the trillions of microorganisms that reside within our digestive system, has emerged as a crucial player in the aging process. Imbalances or disruptions to the gut microbiome have been linked to a wide range of age-related conditions, including metabolic disorders, immune dysfunction, and neurodegenerative diseases.

To support a healthy and resilient gut microbiome, individuals may consider incorporating supplements such as:

- Probiotics: These beneficial bacteria can help restore balance to the gut, support immune function, and potentially promote healthy aging.
  - Prebiotics: Fibers that feed the gut's resident microbes, prebiotics can

help nourish and maintain a diverse, thriving microbiome.

- Postbiotics: The metabolic byproducts of probiotic bacteria, postbiotics have been associated with anti-inflammatory and gut-protective effects.

By nurturing the gut microbiome through the strategic use of these supplements, individuals can support a wide range of physiological processes that are essential for longevity and overall well-being.

Potential Risks and Interactions of Dietary Supplements

While the potential benefits of dietary supplements in the context of anti-aging are compelling, it is crucial to recognize that the use of these products is not without its risks and considerations. Individuals must exercise caution and work closely with healthcare professionals to ensure the safe and effective incorporation of supplements into their longevity regimen.

Quality and Purity Concerns

One of the primary concerns with dietary supplements is the issue of quality and purity. The supplement industry is largely unregulated, and there have been instances of products containing contaminants, adulterants, or undisclosed ingredients that can pose a threat to consumer health.

To mitigate these risks, individuals should prioritize the purchase of supplements from reputable, third-party-tested brands that adhere to good manufacturing practices (GMPs) and provide transparency regarding their ingredient sourcing and testing procedures.

Interactions with Medications and Underlying Conditions

Dietary supplements can also potentially interact with certain medications or exacerbate underlying health conditions. For example, supplements that affect blood clotting, such as ginkgo biloba or fish oil, may interact with anticoagulant or antiplatelet medications, while supplements that influence blood sugar regulation, like chromium or vanadium, may impact the management of diabetes.

Before incorporating any dietary supplements into their longevity regimen, individuals should consult with their healthcare provider, particularly if they are taking prescription medications or have pre-existing medical conditions. This allows for the identification of potential interactions and the development of a personalized supplementation plan that prioritizes safety and effectiveness.

Dosage and Toxicity Concerns

Another important consideration when using dietary supplements is the appropriate dosage and the potential for toxicity. While many supplements are generally well-tolerated at recommended levels, excessive or prolonged consumption can lead to adverse effects, such as liver or kidney damage, gastrointestinal distress, or even an increased risk of certain health conditions.

It is essential for individuals to follow the guidance provided on supplement labels, as well as to work closely with healthcare professionals to determine the optimal dosage based on their specific needs, age, and overall health status. Regular monitoring and adjustments may be necessary to ensure the safe and effective use of supplements over the long term.

Personalized Approach to Supplementation

As with many aspects of the anti-aging journey, the integration of dietary supplements and nutraceuticals into a comprehensive longevity strategy requires a personalized approach that takes into account an individual's unique genetic profile, lifestyle factors, and underlying health conditions.

Genetic and Metabolic Considerations

An individual's genetic makeup can influence their body's absorption, metabolism, and response to various nutrients and bioactive compounds found in dietary supplements. By incorporating genetic testing and personalized biomarker analysis, healthcare professionals can help identify an individual's specific nutritional needs and vulnerabilities, allowing for the development of a tailored supplementation plan.

For example, individuals with certain genetic variants may be predisposed to increased oxidative stress or have a higher requirement for specific antioxidants, such as vitamin C or glutathione. Similarly, genetic factors can influence an individual's response to supplements that target pathways like insulin/IGF-1 signaling or telomere maintenance. By addressing these personalized genetic considerations, individuals can ensure the optimal efficacy and safety of their supplement regimen.

Underlying Health Conditions and Medication Interactions

In addition to genetic factors, an individual's current health status and any underlying medical conditions can also significantly impact their supplementation needs and the potential for adverse interactions.

Individuals with chronic diseases, such as cardiovascular disease, diabetes, or autoimmune disorders, may require specialized supplementation protocols to address their unique physiological challenges and ensure the safe integration of supplements with their existing medications or treatments.

Similarly, individuals who are taking prescription medications should work closely with their healthcare providers to carefully evaluate the potential for supplement-drug interactions and develop a supplementation plan that minimizes the risk of adverse effects.

Ongoing Monitoring and Adjustments

Given the dynamic nature of the aging process and the potential for changes in an individual's health status over time, the personalization of a supplementation regimen must be an ongoing process, with regular monitoring and adjustments as needed.

Healthcare professionals should work closely with individuals to periodically assess the effectiveness and safety of their supplement use, monitoring for any changes in biomarkers, the emergence of new health concerns, or the need to adapt the supplementation plan to align with the individual's evolving needs and priorities.

By embracing a personalized, evidence-based approach to supplementation, individuals can unlock the full potential of these bioactive compounds in the pursuit of healthy longevity, while minimizing the risk of adverse effects and ensuring the long-term sustainability of their anti-aging efforts.

Integrating Supplements into a Comprehensive Anti-Aging Lifestyle

As we have explored throughout this chapter, the strategic use of dietary supplements and nutraceuticals can play a valuable role in supporting the body's natural defenses against the ravages of time. However, it is crucial to recognize that these supplements should not be viewed as a standalone solution, but rather as one component of a comprehensive, holistic approach to anti-aging.

By seamlessly integrating the use of targeted supplements into a broader lifestyle framework that addresses other key aspects of health and longevity, individuals can create a powerful synergistic effect that amplifies the benefits of their anti-aging efforts.

For example, the incorporation of omega-3 supplements to combat inflammation may be more effective when coupled with a nutrient-dense, anti-inflammatory diet, regular physical activity, and stress management techniques. Similarly, the use of adaptogenic herbs to support the body's stress response can be further enhanced by ensuring adequate, high-quality sleep and fostering emotional well-being.

Furthermore, the personalization of a supplementation regimen should be closely aligned with an individual's genetic profile, underlying health conditions, and unique physiological needs. By working closely with healthcare professionals, individuals can develop a tailored plan that not only addresses specific nutritional gaps or age-related challenges but also integrates seamlessly with their broader anti-aging lifestyle.

Embracing the Power of Supplementation in Longevity

As we continue to navigate the complex and ever-evolving landscape of anti-aging, the role of dietary supplements and nutraceuticals emerges as a powerful tool in the pursuit of healthy longevity. By leveraging the latest scientific advancements and the growing body of evidence supporting the benefits of these bioactive compounds, individuals can unlock a new realm of possibilities in their quest for a longer, healthier, and more vibrant life.

However, the true transformative power of supplementation lies not only in its ability to address specific physiological needs but also in its capacity to empower individuals to take a more proactive and personalized approach to their overall health and well-being. By understanding the nuances of their own genetic and metabolic profiles, and by working closely with healthcare professionals to develop a customized supplementation plan, individuals can foster a profound sense of agency and control over their aging trajectory.

As you continue your journey towards longevity, remember that the integration of dietary supplements and nutraceuticals is not a one-size-fits-all proposition. It is a deeply personal and dynamic process that requires a holistic, evidence-based approach, tailored to your unique needs and priorities. By embracing this personalized path, you can unlock the full potential of supplementation, paving the way for a future filled with optimal health, enhanced resilience, and the boundless joy of a life well-lived.

Embark on this transformative journey, where the strategic use of bioactive compounds serves as a vital component of a comprehensive anti-aging strategy. Together, let us unlock the secrets to a longer, healthier, and more vibrant future, one supplement and nutraceutical at a time.

CHAPTER 11

E merging Anti-Aging Therapies

As the scientific and medical communities continue to push the boundaries of longevity research, a new frontier of innovative anti-aging therapies has emerged, offering the promise of unprecedented rejuvenation and the potential to rewrite the narrative of aging. From cutting-edge stem cell therapies to revolutionary gene-based interventions, the landscape of anti-aging is evolving at a rapid pace, providing individuals with a tantalizing glimpse into the future of healthy longevity.

In this chapter, we will explore some of the most promising and transformative anti-aging therapies currently in development, delving into the science behind these innovative approaches and discussing their potential implications for the pursuit of a longer, healthier, and more vibrant life.

Stem Cell Therapies and Regenerative Medicine

One of the most exciting and promising areas of anti-aging research involves the field of stem cell therapies and regenerative medicine. Stem cells, with their remarkable ability to self-renew and differentiate into a wide range of specialized cell types, have emerged as a powerful tool in the quest for cellular rejuvenation and tissue repair.

The Regenerative Potential of Stem Cells

Stem cells, whether derived from embryonic, adult, or induced pluripotent sources, hold the key to unlocking the body's natural capacity for regeneration and repair. These remarkable cells possess the inherent ability to replace damaged or dysfunctional tissues, potentially reversing the effects of aging and age-related diseases.

Some of the ways in which stem cell therapies can contribute to the anti-aging process include:

1. Cellular Rejuvenation: Stem cells can be used to replace or replenish aging or damaged cells, restoring the body's youthful cellular composition and function.

2. Tissue Regeneration: By differentiating into specific cell types, stem cells can help rebuild and repair tissues that have been compromised by the aging process, such as the cardiovascular system, musculoskeletal structure, or the nervous system.

3. Immune System Enhancement: Stem cell-based therapies have the potential to modulate the immune system, strengthening the body's defenses against age-related diseases and supporting overall health and longevity.

4. Organ Regeneration: In the case of organ failure or significant age-related decline, stem cell-derived organoids or bioengineered organs could one day provide a means of replacing and rejuvenating essential bodily systems.

Ongoing Clinical Trials and Emerging Therapies

The promise of stem cell therapies in the field of anti-aging has already sparked a wave of clinical trials and the development of innovative regenerative treatments. Some of the most promising areas of research and development include:

1. Mesenchymal Stem Cell Therapies: These versatile stem cells, often

derived from sources like bone marrow or adipose tissue, are being explored for their potential to combat age-related diseases, such as osteoarthritis, cardiovascular conditions, and neurodegenerative disorders.

2. Induced Pluripotent Stem Cell (iPSC) Therapies: By reprogramming adult cells into a pluripotent state, researchers can create personalized stem cells that can be used for tissue repair and regeneration, potentially addressing the unique needs and vulnerabilities of individual patients.

3. Stem Cell-Derived Organoid Therapies: The use of stem cell-derived organoids, which are miniature, self-organizing organ models, holds the promise of revolutionizing the treatment of age-related organ failure and the replacement of damaged tissues.

4. Exosome-Based Therapies: Exosomes, the tiny vesicles released by stem cells, have been found to carry a wealth of regenerative factors and may offer a novel, cell-free approach to promoting tissue repair and rejuvenation.

As these stem cell-based therapies continue to evolve and progress through clinical trials, they hold the potential to dramatically transform the landscape of anti-aging, offering individuals the opportunity to harness the body's innate regenerative capabilities and combat the ravages of time.

Calorie Restriction and Fasting Mimetics

Another promising area of anti-aging research involves the exploration of calorie restriction and fasting-mimetic compounds, which have been shown to have a profound impact on longevity and healthspan in a wide range of animal models.

The Benefits of Calorie Restriction

Calorie restriction, the practice of reducing overall caloric intake by 10-30% without causing malnutrition, has long been recognized as one of the most effective and well-studied interventions for extending lifespan and promoting healthy aging.

The mechanisms behind calorie restriction's anti-aging effects are multifaceted and involve a complex interplay of cellular and physiological adaptations, including:

1. Reduced Oxidative Stress: Calorie restriction has been shown to lower the production of harmful free radicals and reactive oxygen species, mitigating the detrimental effects of oxidative stress on cellular function and the aging process.

2. Improved Metabolic Efficiency: Calorie restriction can enhance the body's metabolic efficiency, improving glucose and lipid homeostasis, and reducing the risk of age-related metabolic disorders.

3. Modulation of Nutrient-Sensing Pathways: Calorie restriction can favorably regulate key longevity-associated pathways, such as the insulin/IGF-1 signaling and the mechanistic target of rapamycin (mTOR) pathways, which play crucial roles in the aging process.

4. Cellular Stress Resistance: Calorie restriction can activate cellular stress response mechanisms, enhancing the body's ability to cope with and adapt to various stressors, ultimately promoting cellular resilience and longevity.

While the implementation of a calorie-restricted diet can be challenging for many individuals, the exploration of fasting-mimetic compounds has emerged as a promising alternative approach to reaping the anti-aging benefits of calorie restriction.

Fasting Mimetics: Harnessing the Power of Calorie Restriction

Fasting mimetics are a class of compounds that can mimic the physiological effects of calorie restriction or intermittent fasting, without the need for drastic reductions in food intake. These compounds have the potential to provide the longevity-promoting benefits of calorie restriction while being more accessible and sustainable for individuals.

Some of the most widely studied fasting mimetics include:

1. Metformin: This diabetes medication has been shown to have broad-spectrum anti-aging effects, potentially by activating the AMPK pathway and modulating nutrient-sensing mechanisms.

2. Resveratrol: This polyphenol compound, found in red wine and certain berries, has been associated with the activation of longevity-related pathways, such as the SIRT1 gene.

3. Rapamycin: Also known as sirolimus, this immunosuppressant drug has been found to extend lifespan in animal models by inhibiting the mTOR pathway, which plays a crucial role in the aging process.

4. Spermidine: This polyamine compound has been linked to the induction of autophagy, a cellular process that helps remove damaged organelles and proteins, potentially contributing to longevity.

By leveraging the power of these fasting mimetics, individuals can potentially harness the anti-aging benefits of calorie restriction without the need for drastic dietary changes, making this approach more accessible and sustainable in the long term.

Senolytics and Senescent Cell Clearance

Another emerging area of anti-aging research involves the targeting and elimination of senescent cells, which are those that have reached the end of their replicative lifespan and can no longer divide. The accumulation of these senescent cells has been identified as a key hallmark of aging, contributing to the development of various age-related diseases and the overall deterioration of tissue function.

The Burden of Cellular Senescence

As we grow older, our cells gradually accumulate various forms of damage, including DNA damage, telomere attrition, and mitochondrial dysfunction. In response to these stressors, cells can enter a state of permanent cell cycle arrest, known as cellular senescence.

While senescent cells were once essential for growth and development, their persistent presence in aging tissues can have detrimental effects, including:

1. Secretion of Inflammatory Factors: Senescent cells release a range of pro-inflammatory cytokines, chemokines, and other factors, contributing to chronic inflammation and the promotion of age-related diseases.

2. Impaired Tissue Regeneration: The accumulation of senescent cells can disrupt the normal function of stem cells and progenitor cells, impairing the body's ability to repair and rejuvenate tissues.

3. Disruption of Cellular Function: Senescent cells can negatively impact the function of neighboring healthy cells through direct cell-to-cell interactions or the release of harmful secretions.

4. Increased Risk of Age-Related Diseases: The presence of senescent cells has been linked to the development of various age-related conditions, such as cancer, cardiovascular disease, and neurodegenerative disorders.

Senolytics: Selectively Eliminating Senescent Cells

In recognition of the detrimental role that senescent cells play in the aging process, researchers have been exploring the development of senolytic compounds – drugs that can selectively eliminate these harmful cells while leaving healthy cells unharmed.

The selective removal of senescent cells, through the use of senolytics, has been associated with a range of potential anti-aging benefits, including:

1. Improved Tissue Function: The clearance of senescent cells can help restore the normal function of tissues and organs, potentially reversing age-related declines in physical and cognitive performance.

2. Reduced Chronic Inflammation: By removing the source of inflammatory factors, senolytic therapies can help mitigate the damaging effects of chronic inflammation on the aging process.

3. Enhanced Stem Cell Activity: The elimination of senescent cells can create a more permissive environment for the proliferation and differentiation of stem cells, supporting tissue regeneration and repair.

4. Delayed Onset of Age-Related Diseases: Senolytic interventions have shown promise in delaying or preventing the development of various age-related conditions, such as osteoarthritis, pulmonary fibrosis, and neurodegenerative disorders.

While the field of senolytic therapies is still in its early stages, with ongoing clinical trials and further research required, the potential of these interventions to transform the landscape of anti-aging is undeniable.

Emerging Gene-Based Anti-Aging Therapies

As our understanding of the genetic and epigenetic factors that influence the aging process continues to evolve, the exploration of gene-based anti-aging therapies has become an increasingly promising area of research. From the targeted modulation of longevity-associated genes to the development of gene-editing technologies, these innovative approaches hold the promise of directly addressing the molecular underpinnings of aging.

Genetic Interventions for Longevity

One of the key areas of focus in gene-based anti-aging therapies involves the identification and targeted manipulation of specific genes and genetic pathways that have been associated with longevity.

For example, researchers have explored the potential of interventions that target the sirtuins, a family of genes that play crucial roles in regulating cellular processes like DNA repair, metabolism, and stress response – all of which are essential for healthy aging. By developing targeted therapies that can enhance the activity of these longevity-associated genes, researchers aim to directly address the genetic drivers of the aging process.

Similarly, the exploration of gene-based therapies that modulate the insulin/IGF-1 signaling pathway or the mechanistic target of rapamycin (mTOR) pathway, both of which have been linked to lifespan extension in various model organisms, holds promise for the future of anti-aging interventions.

Gene Editing and Epigenetic Modulation

In addition to the targeted manipulation of specific genes, the field of anti-aging research has also been exploring the potential of gene-editing technologies, such as CRISPR-Cas9, to directly address the genetic under-pinnings of aging.

These gene-editing tools offer the possibility of precisely modifying the DNA sequence, allowing for the correction of genetic mutations, the silencing of deleterious genes, or the enhancement of longevity-associated genetic variants. By harnessing the power of gene editing, researchers aim to develop interventions that can directly target and potentially reverse the genetic drivers of the aging process.

Furthermore, the field of epigenetics, which focuses on the dynamic and reversible modifications that influence gene expression without altering the underlying DNA sequence, has also emerged as a promising area of exploration in the context of anti-aging. By developing therapies that can favorably modulate the epigenetic landscape, researchers hope to unlock new avenues for promoting healthy longevity and addressing the complex, multifactorial nature of the aging process.

The Promises and Challenges of Gene-Based Anti-Aging Therapies

The development of gene-based anti-aging therapies holds immense potential, offering the possibility of directly addressing the molecular mechanisms that underpin the aging process. However, the implementation of these innovative approaches also comes with a unique set of challenges and considerations.

Safety and Ethical Concerns: Gene-based interventions, particularly those involving gene editing, raise important safety and ethical concerns, as the long-term consequences of these therapies are not yet fully understood. Rigorous testing and regulatory oversight are essential to ensure the safety and responsible development of these technologies.

Accessibility and Equity: As with many emerging medical innovations, there is a risk that gene-based anti-aging therapies may initially be accessible only to a privileged few, raising concerns about equity and the potential to exacerbate existing health disparities. Ensuring the affordability and widespread availability of these interventions will be a crucial challenge to address.

Personalization and Precision: Given the complex and individualized nature of the aging process, the successful implementation of gene-based anti-aging therapies will require a highly personalized and precision-based approach, taking into account an individual's unique genetic profile, epigenetic landscape, and overall health status.

Ongoing Research and Collaboration

Despite the challenges, the field of gene-based anti-aging therapies continues to evolve rapidly, with researchers and healthcare professionals around the world working tirelessly to unlock the secrets of longevity and develop innovative interventions that can transform the aging experience.

As these cutting-edge therapies progress through clinical trials and regulatory approval processes, it will be essential for individuals to stay informed, engage with healthcare providers, and advocate for the responsible and equitable development of these transformative technologies.

Embracing the Promise of Emerging Anti-Aging Therapies

As we have explored in this chapter, the landscape of anti-aging is undergoing a profound transformation, with the emergence of innovative therapies that hold the promise of unprecedented rejuvenation and the potential to rewrite the narrative of aging.

From the regenerative power of stem cell-based interventions to the targeted elimination of senescent cells and the direct modulation of genetic and epigenetic factors, these cutting-edge approaches have the potential to unlock new frontiers of healthy longevity, empowering individuals to take control of their aging trajectory and unlock the boundless potential of a longer, healthier, and more vibrant life.

However, the true transformative power of these emerging anti-aging therapies lies not only in their ability to combat the ravages of time but also in their capacity to inspire a shift in the collective mindset towards aging. By embracing the promise of these innovative interventions, individuals can foster a profound sense of hope, agency, and optimism, redefining the very notion of what it means to grow older.

As you continue your journey towards longevity, remember that the path ahead is not without its challenges and complexities. Navigating the rapidly evolving landscape of anti-aging therapies will require a deep understanding of the science, a willingness to engage with healthcare professionals, and a steadfast commitment to the responsible and equitable development of these transformative technologies.

Embark on this transformative journey, where the boundaries of what is possible in the realm of aging are continuously redefined. Together, let us unlock the full potential of a future where the ravages of time are not merely accepted, but actively confronted and overcome, paving the way for a new era of vibrant, rejuvenated, and enduring longevity.

CHAPTER 12

Longevity Lifestyle Integration

As we have explored throughout this book, the pursuit of longevity is a multifaceted and deeply personal journey, involving the integration of a comprehensive range of strategies and interventions aimed at slowing the aging process and promoting optimal health and vitality. While the individual components of this anti-aging roadmap – from nutrition and exercise to emerging therapies and personalized approaches – are essential, the true transformative power lies in the seamless integration of these elements into a cohesive, holistic lifestyle.

In this final chapter, we will delve into the art of crafting a comprehensive anti-aging plan that addresses the various facets of the aging experience, empowering you to create a synergistic effect that amplifies the benefits of your longevity efforts and sets you on a path towards a longer, healthier, and more vibrant future.

Creating a Comprehensive Anti-Aging Plan

Embarking on the quest for longevity can feel daunting, with the sheer volume of information and the seemingly endless array of strategies to consider. However, by adopting a systematic and holistic approach, you can develop a comprehensive anti-aging plan that addresses your unique needs, goals, and preferences, setting you up for long-term success.

Step 1: Assess Your Current Health and Lifestyle

The first step in creating your comprehensive anti-aging plan is to take a deep dive into your current health status and lifestyle habits. This assessment should include a thorough evaluation of your:

- Physical health: Measure key biomarkers, such as blood pressure, cholesterol levels, and body composition.
  - Nutritional status: Analyze your dietary intake, identify nutrient deficiencies, and assess your overall eating patterns.
  - Physical activity levels: Evaluate the frequency, duration, and intensity of your exercise routine.
  - Sleep quality and quantity: Monitor your sleep patterns and identify any disruptions or challenges.
  - Stress levels and emotional well-being: Assess your stress management techniques and overall mental health.
  - Genetic and family health history: Understand your predispositions and potential risk factors for age-related diseases.

By gathering this comprehensive baseline data, you can gain a clear understanding of your starting point and identify the specific areas that require the most attention in your anti-aging journey.

Step 2: Establish Your Longevity Goals

With a solid understanding of your current health and lifestyle, the next step is to define your longevity goals. These goals should be specific, measurable, and tailored to your individual needs and aspirations. Some examples of longevity goals may include:

- Maintaining a healthy weight and body composition
  - Improving cardiovascular health and reducing the risk of heart disease
  - Preserving cognitive function and preventing age-related memory loss
  - Enhancing physical strength, flexibility, and mobility
  - Reducing the risk of age-related chronic diseases, such as diabetes or

cancer
  - Achieving a greater sense of emotional well-being and stress resilience
  - Extending your healthy lifespan and delaying the onset of age-related decline

By clearly articulating your longevity goals, you can create a roadmap that aligns your various anti-aging strategies and interventions with your desired outcomes.

Step 3: Develop a Personalized Anti-Aging Lifestyle Plan

With your assessment and goals in place, the next step is to develop a personalized anti-aging lifestyle plan that integrates the key components discussed throughout this book. This comprehensive plan should address the following areas:

Nutrition: Craft a nutrient-dense, anti-inflammatory dietary approach that supports cellular health, reduces oxidative stress, and promotes metabolic balance.

Physical Activity: Incorporate a well-rounded exercise regimen that includes strength training, cardiovascular exercise, and activities that challenge your cognitive function.

Sleep and Circadian Optimization: Implement strategies to ensure adequate, high-quality sleep and align your body's internal clock for optimal hormonal regulation and cellular rejuvenation.

Stress Management and Emotional Well-being: Adopt a range of stress-reducing techniques, such as mindfulness meditation, and cultivate positive emotional states to support overall resilience and longevity.

Hormone Balance: Develop a plan to maintain hormonal equilibrium, addressing any age-related imbalances through lifestyle modifications, targeted supplementation, or hormone replacement therapy (if appropriate).

Genetic and Epigenetic Optimization: Leverage insights from genetic testing and epigenetic profiling to tailor your anti-aging strategies and address your unique vulnerabilities and predispositions.

Supplementation and Nutraceuticals: Incorporate evidence-based dietary supplements and bioactive compounds that can provide targeted support for your longevity goals.

Emerging Therapies: Stay informed about the latest developments in anti-aging therapies, such as stem cell treatments or gene-based interventions, and explore their potential integration into your plan (under the guidance of healthcare professionals).

By weaving these various components into a cohesive, personalized anti-aging lifestyle plan, you can create a synergistic effect that amplifies the benefits of your longevity efforts and sets you on a path towards a longer, healthier, and more vibrant future.

Balancing Different Anti-Aging Strategies

As you navigate the creation of your comprehensive anti-aging plan, it is essential to recognize that the path to longevity is not a one-size-fits-all proposition. Each individual will have unique needs, preferences, and priorities when it comes to the various strategies and interventions they choose to incorporate into their lifestyle.

Balancing the different anti-aging approaches, and finding the right blend that aligns with your individual circumstances, is crucial for ensuring the long-term sustainability and effectiveness of your plan.

Navigating the Tradeoffs and Priorities

When crafting your anti-aging lifestyle plan, you may encounter situations where certain strategies or interventions may conflict with or take precedence over others. For example, the implementation of a highly restrictive calorie-restricted diet may be at odds with your enjoyment of social gatherings and the emotional benefits of shared meals. Similarly, the pursuit of an intensive exercise regimen may need to be balanced with the need for adequate rest and recovery to support cellular rejuvenation.

In these instances, it is important to carefully evaluate the tradeoffs and prioritize the strategies that align most closely with your overall longevity goals and personal preferences. This may involve making informed compromises, such as adopting a more moderate calorie restriction approach or incorporating a mix of high-intensity and lower-intensity physical activities.

By maintaining a flexible and adaptable mindset, you can navigate these tradeoffs and find the right balance that allows you to reap the maximum benefits of your anti-aging efforts while also preserving your quality of life and emotional well-being.

Integrating New Strategies and Interventions

As you progress on your longevity journey, you may encounter emerging therapies, cutting-edge technologies, or novel scientific discoveries that pique your interest and potentially offer additional avenues for optimizing your health and lifespan.

When considering the integration of these new strategies and interventions into your comprehensive anti-aging plan, it is essential to approach them with a critical eye and a deep understanding of the underlying science, potential risks, and long-term implications.

Work closely with your healthcare team to thoroughly evaluate the safety, efficacy, and personalized applicability of any new anti-aging approaches. Carefully weigh the potential benefits against the potential drawbacks, and make informed decisions that align with your values, goals, and overall well-being.

Furthermore, remember that the integration of new strategies should not come at the expense of the foundational lifestyle pillars that have already been established. Maintain a balanced and holistic perspective, ensuring that any new interventions seamlessly complement and enhance your existing anti-aging regimen, rather than disrupt the synergistic effects you have already achieved.

Overcoming Challenges and Maintaining Motivation

As you embark on your comprehensive anti-aging journey, it is essential to recognize that the path ahead may not always be smooth or straightforward. You may encounter various challenges, setbacks, and obstacles that test your resolve and threaten to derail your progress. However, by anticipating these challenges and developing strategies to overcome them, you can maintain the motivation and resilience necessary to achieve your longevity goals.

Navigating Setbacks and Adjusting Your Plan

Throughout your anti-aging journey, you may face setbacks, such as plateauing progress, unexpected health issues, or the inability to adhere to certain lifestyle changes. When these challenges arise, it is important to approach them with an open and adaptable mindset, rather than becoming discouraged or feeling like a failure.

When confronted with setbacks, take the time to carefully evaluate the underlying causes and make the necessary adjustments to your comprehensive anti-aging plan. This may involve re-assessing your goals, troubleshooting specific barriers, or seeking the guidance of healthcare professionals to identify alternative strategies that better suit your current needs and circumstances.

Remember that the path to longevity is not linear, and it is natural to experience ups and downs along the way. By embracing a growth mindset and a willingness to learn from your experiences, you can turn these setbacks into opportunities for growth and refinement, ultimately strengthening your resolve and enhancing the long-term effectiveness of your anti-aging efforts.

Cultivating Sustainable Motivation and Accountability

Maintaining the motivation and discipline required to adhere to a comprehensive anti-aging lifestyle can be a significant challenge, especially in the face of competing priorities, temptations, or the gradual normalization of unhealthy habits.

To foster sustainable motivation, consider the following strategies:

1. Regularly reflect on your "why": Revisit your longevity goals and the deeper personal reasons that drive your pursuit of a longer, healthier life. Connecting with this sense of purpose can help you stay focused and committed during times of difficulty.

2. Celebrate small wins: Acknowledge and celebrate the incremental progress you make, no matter how seemingly insignificant. This can help maintain a positive momentum and reinforce the effectiveness of your efforts.

3. Enlist a support network: Surround yourself with like-minded individuals, whether it's family, friends, or a community of health-conscious individuals, who can provide encouragement, accountability, and a shared sense of purpose.

4. Incorporate enjoyable activities: Ensure that your anti-aging lifestyle includes elements that you genuinely enjoy, whether it's a favorite physical activity, a delicious and nourishing meal, or a relaxing self-care routine. This can help prevent burnout and maintain your enthusiasm over the long term.

5. Regularly review and adjust your plan: Periodically revisit your compre-

hensive anti-aging plan, evaluating its effectiveness and making any necessary adjustments to keep it aligned with your evolving needs and preferences.

By cultivating sustainable motivation and accountability, you can navigate the challenges and complexities of your longevity journey with resilience, determination, and a deep sense of purpose.

Embracing the Transformative Power of Longevity Lifestyle Integration

As you reach the culmination of your journey through this comprehensive anti-aging guide, it becomes clear that the true power of longevity lies not in the pursuit of isolated strategies or interventions, but rather in the seamless integration of a diverse range of approaches into a cohesive, holistic lifestyle.

By crafting a personalized anti-aging plan that addresses the multifaceted nature of the aging process, you unlock a synergistic potential that amplifies the benefits of your efforts and sets you on a path towards a longer, healthier, and more vibrant future.

This transformative power of longevity lifestyle integration extends far beyond the physical aspects of health and well-being. By cultivating a deep understanding of the various factors that influence the aging process, and by developing the resilience and adaptability to navigate the inevitable challenges that arise, you can foster a profound sense of empowerment, agency, and control over your own life trajectory.

Moreover, the embrace of a comprehensive anti-aging lifestyle can have a ripple effect, positively impacting not only your personal well-being but also the lives of those around you. By setting an example of proactive health and longevity, you can inspire others to embark on their own transformative journeys, contributing to the creation of a society that values the preservation of health, vitality, and the boundless potential of the human experience.

As you reach the conclusion of this book, remember that the path to longevity is not a destination, but rather a lifelong journey of continuous learning, adaptation, and self-discovery. Embrace the challenges, celebrate the victories, and never lose sight of the profound impact that your personal choices and lifestyle can have on the quality and duration of your life.

Embark on this transformative quest, where the integration of diverse anti-aging strategies serves as the foundation for a future filled with vibrant health, boundless energy, and the profound joy of a life well-lived. Together, let us unlock the full potential of longevity, redefining the very essence of aging and empowering ourselves, and those around us, to embrace the promise of a rejuvenated, enduring, and boundlessly fulfilling existence.

CHAPTER 13

Anti-Aging for Specific Demographics

As we navigate the complex and ever-evolving landscape of anti-aging, it becomes increasingly clear that a one-size-fits-all approach is not the answer. The aging process is a highly individualized experience, shaped by a multitude of factors, including genetic predisposition, environmental influences, and unique physiological characteristics.

In this chapter, we will explore the nuances of anti-aging strategies and considerations for specific demographic groups, recognizing that the path to longevity and optimal health may differ based on an individual's age, gender, and other unique factors. By delving into these specialized approaches, we can empower readers to tailor their anti-aging efforts to their specific needs and unlock the full potential of a longer, healthier, and more vibrant life.

Anti-Aging for Men

While the fundamental principles of anti-aging apply to individuals of all genders, men often face unique challenges and considerations when it comes to maintaining optimal health and vitality as they grow older.

Hormonal Changes and Testosterone Decline

One of the primary concerns for men in the context of anti-aging is the gradual decline in testosterone production, a condition known as andropause or late-onset hypogonadism. As men age, their testosterone levels can steadily decrease, leading to a range of age-related symptoms, such as decreased muscle mass, reduced libido, and impaired sexual function.

To address this hormonal shift, men may consider strategies such as:

- Optimizing their lifestyle factors, including a nutrient-dense diet, regular exercise, and stress management, to support natural testosterone production.
- Exploring the potential benefits of testosterone replacement therapy under the guidance of a healthcare professional, carefully weighing the risks and potential benefits.
- Incorporating supplements that may help maintain healthy testosterone levels, such as zinc, vitamin D, or certain herbal remedies.

Prostate Health and Urological Concerns

As men age, they also face an increased risk of prostate-related issues, such as benign prostatic hyperplasia (BPH) and prostate cancer. Maintaining prostate health is, therefore, a crucial consideration in the context of male anti-aging.

Strategies to support prostate health may include:

- Regular prostate screenings and examinations to detect any abnormalities or changes early on.
- Incorporating a diet rich in antioxidants, such as lycopene from tomatoes, and anti-inflammatory nutrients to support prostate function.
- Exploring the potential benefits of supplements like saw palmetto or beta-sitosterol, which have been studied for their ability to support prostate health.
- Maintaining a healthy weight and engaging in regular physical activity, as obesity and sedentary lifestyle have been linked to an increased risk of prostate issues.

Cardiovascular Health and Metabolic Considerations

Men are often more susceptible to age-related cardiovascular diseases and metabolic disorders, such as heart disease, stroke, and type 2 diabetes. Addressing these specific health concerns is crucial for promoting longevity in the male population.

Strategies to support cardiovascular and metabolic health may include:

- Adopting a heart-healthy diet rich in whole, unprocessed foods, with a focus on omega-3 fatty acids, antioxidants, and fiber.

- Engaging in regular aerobic exercise and strength training to maintain optimal cardiovascular function and muscle mass.

- Monitoring and managing risk factors, such as high blood pressure, elevated cholesterol, and blood sugar imbalances, through lifestyle modifications and, if necessary, targeted medical interventions.

- Exploring the potential benefits of supplements like omega-3s, CoQ10, or metformin (under medical supervision) to support cardiovascular and metabolic health.

Anti-Aging for Women

While men face their own unique challenges in the context of anti-aging, women also confront distinct considerations and requirements as they navigate the complexities of the aging process.

Hormonal Changes and Menopause

One of the most significant events in a woman's life is the onset of menopause, marked by a significant decline in the production of estrogen and other sex hormones. This hormonal shift can have a profound impact on a woman's physical and emotional well-being, contributing to a range of age-related symptoms, such as hot flashes, vaginal dryness, and mood changes.

To address the challenges of menopause and support overall hormonal health, women may consider strategies such as:

- Adopting a diet rich in phytoestrogens, such as soy, flaxseed, and legumes, which may help alleviate menopausal symptoms.
    - Exploring the potential benefits of hormone replacement therapy (HRT) under the guidance of a healthcare provider, carefully weighing the risks and benefits.
    - Incorporating mind-body practices like yoga, meditation, or cognitive-behavioral therapy to manage stress and support emotional well-being.
    - Maintaining regular physical activity, as exercise has been shown to help mitigate the effects of hormonal changes on the body.

Bone Health and Osteoporosis
    Women are at a higher risk of developing osteoporosis, a condition characterized by the gradual loss of bone density and strength. This increased susceptibility is largely due to the hormonal changes associated with menopause, which can accelerate the loss of bone mass.

To support bone health and reduce the risk of osteoporosis, women may consider strategies such as:

- Ensuring adequate intake of calcium, vitamin D, and other bone-supportive nutrients through diet and supplementation.
    - Engaging in weight-bearing exercises and strength training to promote the maintenance of bone density.
    - Exploring the potential benefits of medications like bisphosphonates or selective estrogen receptor modulators (SERMs), under medical supervision, to prevent or manage osteoporosis.
    - Maintaining a healthy lifestyle, including the avoidance of smoking and excessive alcohol consumption, which can further compromise bone health.

Breast Health and Cancer Prevention

Women also face an increased risk of certain age-related cancers, particularly breast cancer, which becomes more prevalent as they grow older. Maintaining optimal breast health and implementing preventive strategies are crucial for women's longevity.

Strategies to support breast health and cancer prevention may include:

- Adherence to recommended breast cancer screening guidelines, such as regular mammograms and self-examinations.
   - Adopting a nutrient-dense, anti-inflammatory diet that includes breast-protective foods like cruciferous vegetables, berries, and healthy fats.
   - Engaging in regular physical activity, as exercise has been associated with a reduced risk of breast cancer.
   - Exploring the potential benefits of supplements like vitamin D, omega-3 fatty acids, or green tea extract, which have been studied for their potential cancer-preventive properties.

Anti-Aging for Older Adults

As individuals continue to age, the specific challenges and considerations in the pursuit of longevity become increasingly nuanced and complex. Older adults face a unique set of physiological, cognitive, and social changes that require a tailored approach to anti-aging strategies.

Sarcopenia and Muscle Maintenance
   One of the hallmarks of aging is the gradual loss of muscle mass and strength, a condition known as sarcopenia. This age-related decline in muscle function can have a significant impact on an older adult's physical independence, mobility, and overall quality of life.

To combat sarcopenia and maintain muscle health, older adults may consider strategies such as:

- Engaging in regular resistance training and strength-building exercises, tailored to their individual physical abilities and limitations.

- Ensuring adequate protein intake, potentially with the support of protein supplements, to support muscle growth and repair.

- Exploring the potential benefits of supplements like creatine, beta-alanine, or specific amino acids, which have been studied for their ability to support muscle health in older adults.

- Addressing any underlying health conditions or nutritional deficiencies that may contribute to the deterioration of muscle mass and function.

Cognitive Decline and Brain Health

As individuals grow older, they also face an increased risk of age-related cognitive decline and the development of neurodegenerative diseases, such as Alzheimer's and Parkinson's. Maintaining brain health and cognitive function is, therefore, a crucial priority for older adults.

Strategies to support cognitive health may include:

- Engaging in regular physical and cognitive exercises, such as puzzles, memory games, or learning new skills, to stimulate the brain and promote neuroplasticity.

- Adopting a nutrient-dense, anti-inflammatory diet rich in antioxidants, omega-3 fatty acids, and other brain-supportive nutrients.

- Exploring the potential benefits of supplements like omega-3s, B vitamins, or herbal remedies, which have been studied for their potential to support cognitive function.

- Addressing underlying health conditions, such as hypertension or diabetes, that can contribute to cognitive decline.

Social Engagement and Emotional Well-being

In addition to the physical and cognitive changes associated with aging, older adults also face unique social and emotional challenges that can impact their overall well-being and longevity.

Strategies to support social engagement and emotional well-being may include:

- Fostering meaningful social connections through participation in community activities, social clubs, or volunteer work.
    - Engaging in mind-body practices like meditation, yoga, or tai chi, which can help manage stress, reduce isolation, and promote emotional resilience.
    - Seeking support from mental health professionals or joining support groups to address any age-related mental health concerns, such as depression or anxiety.
    - Maintaining an active lifestyle and engaging in hobbies or activities that provide a sense of purpose and fulfillment.

Anti-Aging for Younger Individuals

While the focus of anti-aging efforts often centers on older adults, the principles of healthy longevity are equally applicable to younger individuals. In fact, the implementation of proactive anti-aging strategies at an earlier stage in life can have a profound impact on an individual's long-term health and vitality.

Preventive Strategies for the Young

For younger individuals, the focus of anti-aging efforts should be on preventive measures that lay the foundation for a lifetime of optimal health and longevity. This may include strategies such as:

- Adopting a nutrient-dense, anti-inflammatory diet that supports cellular function and metabolic health.
    - Engaging in regular physical activity, including a balance of cardiovascular, strength-building, and mind-body exercises.
    - Prioritizing sleep hygiene and optimizing circadian rhythms to support overall physiological function.
    - Implementing effective stress management techniques, such as mindful-

ness meditation or yoga, to build emotional resilience.
   - Maintaining regular check-ups and screenings to identify any potential health concerns or risk factors early on.

By instilling these healthy habits and preventive measures at a young age, individuals can proactively mitigate the risk of age-related diseases and create a strong foundation for a longer, healthier life.

Addressing Unique Needs and Concerns
   While the core principles of anti-aging apply across all age groups, younger individuals may also face unique needs and concerns that require specialized attention. Some examples include:

- Fertility and reproductive health: Younger individuals may need to consider the impact of certain anti-aging strategies on fertility and reproductive function.
   - Skin health and appearance: Younger individuals may be more focused on maintaining youthful skin and addressing concerns like acne, sun damage, or premature wrinkles.
   - Career and work-life balance: Younger individuals may need to balance their anti-aging efforts with the demands of their professional lives and personal responsibilities.

By addressing these unique needs and concerns, healthcare professionals can help younger individuals develop a comprehensive anti-aging plan that is tailored to their specific stage of life and personal priorities.

Tailoring Anti-Aging Approaches

As we have explored throughout this chapter, the pursuit of longevity and optimal health is not a one-size-fits-all proposition. Each demographic group, from men and women to older adults and younger individuals, faces its own set of challenges and considerations when it comes to the implementation of effective anti-aging strategies.

To ensure the long-term success and sustainability of an individual's anti-aging journey, it is essential to adopt a highly personalized and tailored approach that takes into account the unique characteristics, needs, and vulnerabilities of the specific demographic group.

This personalized approach may involve the following key considerations:

1. Targeted Nutritional and Supplementation Strategies
   Adjusting the dietary recommendations and supplementation protocols to address the specific nutritional requirements and hormonal changes experienced by each demographic group.

2. Customized Exercise and Physical Activity Regimens
   Designing exercise programs that account for the physical capabilities, limitations, and functional goals of the individual, whether they are a young adult, a middle-aged individual, or an older adult.

3. Specialized Screening and Monitoring
   Implementing targeted screening and monitoring protocols to identify potential health concerns or risk factors that are more prevalent in specific demographic groups, such as prostate health in men or bone density in postmenopausal women.

4. Tailored Stress Management and Emotional Support
   Addressing the unique emotional and psychological needs of each demographic group, whether it's navigating the hormonal changes of menopause, the social isolation experienced by older adults, or the work-life balance challenges faced by younger individuals.

5. Integrative and Multidisciplinary Approach
   Collaborating with a diverse team of healthcare professionals, including

physicians, nutritionists, exercise specialists, mental health practitioners, and integrative medicine experts, to ensure a comprehensive and personalized approach to anti-aging.

By embracing this tailored and multifaceted approach to anti-aging, individuals can unlock the full potential of their longevity journey, addressing their specific needs and vulnerabilities while also leveraging the synergistic benefits of a holistic, personalized plan.

Empowering Individuals to Embrace Longevity

As we reach the conclusion of this comprehensive anti-aging guide, the overarching theme that emerges is the profound power of empowerment – the ability of individuals to take control of their own aging trajectory and unlock the secrets to a longer, healthier, and more vibrant life.

Throughout this book, we have explored a diverse range of anti-aging strategies and interventions, from the foundational pillars of nutrition, exercise, and stress management to the cutting-edge frontiers of stem cell therapies, gene-based modifications, and personalized approaches. However, the true transformative power lies not just in the individual components, but in the seamless integration of these elements into a comprehensive, holistic, and tailored anti-aging lifestyle.

By empowering individuals to assess their unique needs, define their longevity goals, and craft a personalized plan that addresses the multifaceted nature of the aging process, we have sought to instill a profound sense of agency and control over one's own health and well-being. This shift in mindset is crucial, as it allows individuals to move beyond passive acceptance of the ravages of time and instead embrace the proactive pursuit of optimal longevity.

Moreover, this empowerment extends beyond the individual, as the widespread adoption of comprehensive anti-aging strategies can have a ripple effect, inspiring positive changes within families, communities, and even society as a whole. By setting an example of proactive health and longevity, individuals can contribute to the creation of a culture that values the preservation of vitality, the cultivation of resilience, and the boundless potential of the human experience.

As you, the reader, embark on your own longevity journey, remember that the path ahead is not a solitary one. Surround yourself with a supportive network of healthcare professionals, like-minded individuals, and a community that shares your passion for healthy aging. Engage in open dialogues, seek out new sources of information, and remain adaptable to the ever-evolving landscape of anti-aging – for the pursuit of longevity is not a destination, but rather a lifelong odyssey of continuous learning, growth, and self-discovery.

Embrace the transformative power of empowerment, and unlock the full potential of a life well-lived. Together, let us redefine the very essence of aging, championing a future where the ravages of time are not merely accepted, but actively confronted and overcome, paving the way for a new era of vibrant, rejuvenated, and enduring longevity.

CONCLUSION

onclusion and Future Outlook

As we reach the culmination of our journey through the vast and ever-evolving landscape of anti-aging, it is essential to take a moment to reflect on the key principles and takeaways that have been woven throughout the pages of this comprehensive guide. Moreover, it is crucial to look towards the future, anticipating the exciting advancements and innovations that hold the promise of transforming the very nature of aging and empowering individuals to unlock the secrets to a longer, healthier, and more vibrant life.

In this final chapter, we will synthesize the core lessons and strategies that have been explored, providing you with a concise and actionable roadmap to guide your ongoing pursuit of longevity. We will also delve into the future outlook of the anti-aging field, offering a glimpse into the cutting-edge developments and emerging therapies that have the potential to rewrite the narrative of aging and redefine the very essence of what it means to grow older.

Summarizing Key Principles and Takeaways

Throughout the course of this book, we have explored a comprehensive range of strategies and interventions aimed at combating the ravages of time and promoting optimal health and vitality. As we reflect on this journey, several key principles and takeaways emerge as the cornerstones of a successful anti-aging approach.

1. Embrace a Holistic and Personalized Mindset

The pursuit of longevity is not a one-size-fits-all proposition. Each individual's path to healthy aging is shaped by a unique combination of genetic, environmental, and lifestyle factors. By adopting a holistic and personalized mindset, you can tailor your anti-aging strategies to address your specific needs, vulnerabilities, and goals, unlocking the full potential of your longevity efforts.

2. Prioritize Lifestyle Modifications

While emerging therapies and cutting-edge interventions hold great promise, the foundation of any successful anti-aging strategy lies in the adoption of evidence-based lifestyle modifications. By optimizing your nutrition, physical activity, sleep, stress management, and emotional well-being, you can create a powerful synergistic effect that supports cellular health, reduces the pace of aging, and promotes overall longevity.

3. Harness the Power of Genetic and Epigenetic Factors

The fields of genomics and epigenetics have revolutionized our understanding of the aging process, revealing the critical role that our genetic makeup and dynamic epigenetic modifications play in shaping our longevity trajectory. By leveraging personalized insights into your genetic and epigenetic profile, you can develop targeted interventions that address the underlying molecular mechanisms driving the aging process.

4. Embrace a Proactive and Preventive Mindset

Rather than passively accepting the ravages of time, adopt a proactive and preventive mindset in your pursuit of longevity. By implementing comprehensive strategies at an earlier stage in life, you can lay the foundation for a lifetime of optimal health and vitality, mitigating the risk of age-related diseases and preserving your independence and quality of life.

5. Cultivate Resilience and Adaptability

The path to longevity is not a linear one; it is filled with challenges, setbacks, and the need for continuous learning and adaptation. By cultivating a resilient mindset and the willingness to adjust your strategies as your needs and circumstances evolve, you can navigate the complexities of the aging process with determination, optimism, and a deep sense of personal agency.

6. Leverage the Power of Community and Collaboration

Your longevity journey is not a solitary endeavor. By surrounding yourself with a supportive network of healthcare professionals, family members, and like-minded individuals, you can foster a sense of accountability, shared experiences, and mutual inspiration – all of which can amplify the effectiveness of your anti-aging efforts.

By embracing these key principles and weaving them into the fabric of your everyday life, you can unlock the transformative power of longevity and embark on a path towards a longer, healthier, and more vibrant future.

Anticipating Future Advancements in Anti-Aging

As we look towards the horizon, the field of anti-aging is poised to undergo a profound transformation, with a myriad of exciting advancements and innovations on the cusp of revolutionizing the way we approach the aging process.

Stem Cell Therapies and Regenerative Medicine

The remarkable potential of stem cells to replace damaged or dysfunctional tissues, as well as the broader field of regenerative medicine, hold the promise of unlocking unprecedented levels of cellular rejuvenation and tissue repair. In the coming years, we can expect to see continued progress in the development of stem cell-based therapies that can address a wide range of age-related conditions, from cardiovascular disease to neurodegenerative disorders.

As these innovative treatments progress through clinical trials and gain regulatory approval, they have the potential to dramatically alter the trajectory of the aging process, empowering individuals to reverse the effects of time and reclaim their physical and cognitive vitality.

Gene-Based Interventions and Epigenetic Modulation

The rapid advancements in our understanding of the genetic and epigenetic factors that influence the aging process have paved the way for the development of highly targeted, gene-based interventions. From the precise editing of longevity-associated genes to the favorable manipulation of the epigenetic landscape, these innovative therapies hold the promise of directly addressing the molecular underpinnings of aging.

In the years ahead, we can anticipate the emergence of increasingly sophisticated gene-based technologies, such as advanced CRISPR-Cas9 systems and targeted epigenetic modulators, that can be tailored to an individual's unique genetic profile and epigenetic vulnerabilities. These transformative interventions have the potential to rewrite the very script of aging, ushering in a new era of personalized, precision-based anti-aging approaches.

Artificial Intelligence and Machine Learning

The integration of artificial intelligence (AI) and machine learning (ML) into the field of anti-aging is poised to revolutionize the way we approach the complexities of the aging process. These powerful technologies can be leveraged to analyze vast troves of data, from an individual's genetic and epigenetic profile to their comprehensive health history and lifestyle factors, to develop highly personalized anti-aging strategies and predict the trajectory of their longevity.

Moreover, AI and ML can also play a crucial role in accelerating the discovery and development of novel anti-aging interventions, from the identification of promising drug candidates to the optimization of existing therapies. As these technologies continue to evolve, we can expect to see the emergence of increasingly sophisticated, data-driven approaches to the pursuit of healthy longevity.

Biotechnology and Nanotechnology

The rapid advancements in the fields of biotechnology and nanotechnology have the potential to dramatically transform the landscape of anti-aging. From the development of nanoscale devices and sensors that can monitor and regulate physiological processes to the engineering of biomimetic materials that can enhance tissue regeneration, these cutting-edge technologies hold the promise of unlocking new frontiers in the quest for longevity.

In the coming years, we can anticipate the emergence of innovative biotechnological solutions, such as smart drug delivery systems, personalized organ printing, and advanced biomonitoring platforms, that can provide unprecedented precision and targeted interventions to combat the ravages of time. As these technologies mature and become more accessible, they can profoundly impact the way we approach the aging process and empower individuals to take control of their longevity.

Integrated, Holistic Approaches

While the individual advancements in areas like stem cell therapies, gene-based interventions, and AI-driven technologies hold immense promise, the true transformative power of the future of anti-aging will likely lie in the seamless integration of these diverse approaches into comprehensive, holistic strategies.

By leveraging the synergistic benefits of cutting-edge interventions, personalized lifestyle modifications, and data-driven insights, the anti-aging solutions of the future will be designed to address the multifaceted nature of the aging process in a highly individualized and optimized manner. This integrated approach will empower individuals to tailor their longevity efforts to their unique genetic predispositions, environmental factors, and personal preferences, unlocking the full potential of a longer, healthier, and more vibrant life.

Empowering Readers to Embrace Longevity

As we reach the culmination of our journey through this comprehensive anti-aging guide, it is clear that the pursuit of longevity is not merely a quest for the extension of lifespan, but a transformative process that has the power to enrich every facet of an individual's life.

Throughout the pages of this book, we have sought to empower you, the reader, with the knowledge, tools, and strategies necessary to take control of your own aging trajectory and unlock the secrets to a longer, healthier, and more vibrant future. From the foundational pillars of lifestyle modification to the cutting-edge frontiers of emerging therapies, we have explored a diverse range of approaches, each one designed to address the multifaceted nature of the aging process and help you achieve your longevity goals.

As you move forward on this transformative journey, remember that the path ahead is not a solitary one. Surround yourself with a supportive network of healthcare professionals, like-minded individuals, and a community that shares your passion for healthy aging. Engage in open dialogues, seek out new sources of information, and remain adaptable to the ever-evolving landscape of anti-aging – for the pursuit of longevity is not a destination, but rather a lifelong odyssey of continuous learning, growth, and self-discovery.

Embrace the power of empowerment, and unlock the full potential of a life well-lived. By taking an active role in shaping your own aging trajectory, you not only reap the benefits of a longer, healthier life but also contribute to the creation of a society that values the preservation of vitality, the cultivation of resilience, and the boundless promise of the human experience.

Together, let us redefine the very essence of aging, championing a future where the ravages of time are not merely accepted, but actively confronted and overcome. Let us unlock the transformative power of longevity, paving the way for a new era of vibrant, rejuvenated, and enduring lives that inspire and uplift not only ourselves but also the world around us.

So, embark on this final chapter of your anti-aging journey with a renewed sense of purpose, determination, and the unwavering belief that the secrets to a longer, healthier life are within your grasp. The future of anti-aging is bright, and the promise of a tomorrow filled with boundless vitality and the joyful celebration of every precious moment is ours to pursue.

www.ingramcontent.com/pod-product-compliance
Lightning Source LLC
Chambersburg PA
CBHW070842250726
48662CB00003B/1329